LARGE-SCALE
BIOMEDICAL SCIENCE

EXPLORING STRATEGIES FOR FUTURE RESEARCH

Committee on Large-Scale Science and Cancer Research
Sharyl J. Nass and Bruce W. Stillman, *Editors*

National Cancer Policy Board

INSTITUTE OF MEDICINE
OF THE NATIONAL ACADEMIES

and

Division on Earth and Life Studies

NATIONAL RESEARCH COUNCIL
OF THE NATIONAL ACADEMIES

THE NATIONAL ACADEMIES
Washington, D.C.
www.nap.edu

THE NATIONAL ACADEMIES PRESS • 500 Fifth Street, N.W. • Washington, DC 20001

NOTICE: The project that is the subject of this report was approved by the Governing Board of the National Research Council, whose members are drawn from the councils of the National Academy of Sciences, the National Academy of Engineering, and the Institute of Medicine. The members of the committee responsible for the report were chosen for their special competences and with regard for appropriate balance.

Support for this project was provided by The National Cancer Institute. The views presented in this report are those of the Institute of Medicine and National Research Council Committee on Large-Scale Science and Cancer Research and are not necessarily those of the funding agencies.

Library of Congress Cataloging-in-Publication Data

Large-scale biomedical science : exploring strategies for future research / Sharyl J. Nass and Bruce W. Stillman, editors ; Committee on Large-scale Science and Cancer Research, National Cancer Policy Board and Division on Earth and Life Studies, National Research Council.
    p. ; cm.
Includes bibliographical references.
 ISBN 0-309-08912-3 (pbk.) — ISBN 0-309-50698-0 (PDF)
 1. Medicine—Research—Government policy—United States. 2. Cancer—Research—Government policy—United States. 3. Federal aid to medical research—United States.
 [DNLM: 1. Biomedical Research—United States. 2. Interinstitutional Relations—United States. 3. Research Design—United States. 4. Resource Allocation—United States. W 20.5 L322 2003] I. Nass, Sharyl J. II. Stillman, Bruce. III. National Cancer Policy Board (U.S.). Committee on Large-scale Science and Cancer Research. IV. National Research Council (U.S.). Division on Earth and Life Studies.
 R854.U5L37 2003
 610'.7'2073—dc21
                    2003009162

Additional copies of this report are available from the National Academies Press, 500 Fifth Street, N.W., Lockbox 285, Washington, DC 20055; (800) 624-6242 or (202) 334-3313 (in the Washington metropolitan area); Internet, http://www.nap.edu.

For more information about the Institute of Medicine, visit the IOM home page at: **www. iom.edu.**

THE NATIONAL ACADEMIES
Advisers to the Nation on Science, Engineering, and Medicine

The **National Academy of Sciences** is a private, nonprofit, self-perpetuating society of distinguished scholars engaged in scientific and engineering research, dedicated to the furtherance of science and technology and to their use for the general welfare. Upon the authority of the charter granted to it by the Congress in 1863, the Academy has a mandate that requires it to advise the federal government on scientific and technical matters. Dr. Bruce M. Alberts is president of the National Academy of Sciences.

The **National Academy of Engineering** was established in 1964, under the charter of the National Academy of Sciences, as a parallel organization of outstanding engineers. It is autonomous in its administration and in the selection of its members, sharing with the National Academy of Sciences the responsibility for advising the federal government. The National Academy of Engineering also sponsors engineering programs aimed at meeting national needs, encourages education and research, and recognizes the superior achievements of engineers. Dr. Wm. A. Wulf is president of the National Academy of Engineering.

The **Institute of Medicine** was established in 1970 by the National Academy of Sciences to secure the services of eminent members of appropriate professions in the examination of policy matters pertaining to the health of the public. The Institute acts under the responsibility given to the National Academy of Sciences by its congressional charter to be an adviser to the federal government and, upon its own initiative, to identify issues of medical care, research, and education. Dr. Harvey V. Fineberg is president of the Institute of Medicine.

The **National Research Council** was organized by the National Academy of Sciences in 1916 to associate the broad community of science and technology with the Academy's purposes of furthering knowledge and advising the federal government. Functioning in accordance with general policies determined by the Academy, the Council has become the principal operating agency of both the National Academy of Sciences and the National Academy of Engineering in providing services to the government, the public, and the scientific and engineering communities. The Council is administered jointly by both Academies and the Institute of Medicine. Dr. Bruce M. Alberts and Dr. Wm. A. Wulf are chair and vice chair, respectively, of the National Research Council.

www.national-academies.org

v

REVIEWERS

This report has been reviewed in draft form by individuals chosen for their diverse perspectives and technical expertise, in accordance with procedures approved by the NRC's Report Review Committee. The purpose of this independent review is to provide candid and critical comments that will assist the institution in making its published report as sound as possible and to ensure that the report meets institutional standards for objectivity, evidence, and responsiveness to the study charge. The review comments and draft manuscript remain confidential to protect the integrity of the deliberative process. We wish to thank the following individuals for their review of this report:

Mina J. Bissell, Ph.D. Distinguished Scientist, Life Sciences Division, Lawrence Berkeley National Laboratory

Marvin Cassman, Ph.D. Director, QB3 at University of California, San Francisco

Mildred Cho, Ph.D. Senior Research Scholar and Acting Co-director, Stanford Center for Biomedical Ethics

Carol Dahl, Ph.D. Biospect, Inc.

Chi Dang, M.D., Ph.D. Professor, Division of Hematology, Johns Hopkins University Department of Medicine

Alfred G. Gilman, M.D., Ph.D. Regental Professor and Chairman, Department of Pharmocology, University of Texas Southwestern Medical Center

Allen S. Lichter, M.D. Newman Family Professor of Radiation Oncology, Dean, University of Michigan Medical School

Candace Swimmer, Ph.D. Research Fellow, Department of Genome Biochemistry, Exelixis, Inc.

Shirley M. Tilghman, Ph.D. President, Princeton University

Although the reviewers listed above have provided many constructive comments and suggestions, they were not asked to endorse the conclusions or recommendations nor did they see the final draft of the report before its release. The review of this report was overseen by **Enriqueta C. Bond, Ph.D., President, Burroughs Wellcome Fund** and **Charles E. Phelps, Ph.D., Provost University of Rochester.** Appointed by the National Research Council and Institute of Medicine, they were responsible for making certain that an independent examination of this report was carried out in accordance with institutional procedures and that all review comments were carefully considered. Responsibility for the final content of this report rests entirely with the authoring committee and the institution.

Acknowledgments

The committee gratefully acknowledges the contributions of many individuals who provided invaluable information and data for the study, either through formal presentations or through informal contacts with the study staff:

Herman Alvarado, Bi Ade, Lee Babiss, Wendy Baldwin, John Carney, Robert Cook-Deegan, Carol Dahl, James Deatherage, Joseph DeRisi, Marie Freire, Jack Gibbons, John Gohagan, Eric Green, Judith Greenberg, Edward Hackett, Edward Harlow, Nathaniel Heintz, David Hirsh, Nancy Hopkins, James Jensen, Marvin Kalt, Richard Klausner, William Koster, Rolph Leming, Joan Leonard, Arnold Levine, David Livingston, Rochelle Long, David Longfellow, Michael Lorenz, Richard Lyttle, Pamela Marino, Richard Nelson, Emanuel Petricoin, Michael Rogers, Jacques Rossouw, Walter Schaefer, William Schraeder, Stuart Schreiber, Edward Scolnick, Scott Somers, Paula Stephan, Marcus Stoffel, Robert Strausberg, Daniel Sullivan, Roy Vagelos, Craig Venter, LeRoy Walters, Barbara Weber, Michael Wigler, Robert Wittes.

Acronyms

AAAS – American Association for the Advancement of Science
AEC – Atomic Energy Commission (forerunner of DOE)
AFCS – Alliance for Cellular Signaling
AIP – American Institute of Physics
AUTM – Association of University Technology Managers

BAA – Broad Agency Announcement

CDC – Centers for Disease Control and Prevention
CEPH – Centre d'Etude du Polymorphisme Humaine
CERN – Conseil European Pour La Rechierche Nucleaire
CES – Cooperative Extension Services
CGAP – Cancer Genome Anatomy Project
COSEPUP – Committee on Science, Engineering, and Public Policy
CRADA – Cooperative Research and Development Agreement
CSR – Center for Scientific Review

DARPA – The Defense Advanced Research Projects Agency
DHHS – Department of Health and Human Services
DOD – Department of Defense
DOE – Department of Energy
DTP – Developmental Therapeutics Program

EDRN – The Early Detection Research Network
EPA – Environmental Protection Agency
EST – Expressed Sequence Tag

FDA – Food and Drug Administration

GPRA – Government Performance and Results Act

HGP – Human Genome Project
HHMI – Howard Hughes Medical Institute
HRT – Hormone Replacement Therapy
HUGO - Human Genome Organization
HUPO – Human Proteome Organization

INS – Immigration and Naturalization Service
IRG – Integrated Review Groups
IUPAP – International Union of Pure and Applied Physics

JCSG – Joint Center for Structure Genomics

MBL – Marine Biology Laboratory
MMHCC – Mouse Models of Human Cancers Consortium
MOU – Memoranda of Understanding

NACA – National Advisory Committee for Aeronautics
NAS – National Academy of Sciences
NASA – National Aeronautics and Space Administration
NCAB – National Cancer Advisory Board
NCI – National Cancer Institute
NDRC – National Defense Research Committee
NHGRI – National Human Genome Research Institute
NHLBI – National Heart Lung and Blood Institute
NIAID – National Institute of Allergy and Infectious Diseases
NIEHS – National Institute of Environmental Health Science
NIGMS – National Institute of General Medical Sciences
NIH – National Institutes of Health
NOAA – National Oceanic and Atmospheric Administration
NOARL – Naval Oceanographic and Atmospheric Research Laboratory
NRAC – Naval Research Advisory Committee
NRC – National Research Council
NRSA – National Research Service Awards
NSF – National Science Foundation
NTP – National Toxicology Program

OES – Office of Experiment Stations
OMB – Office of Management and Budget
ONR – Office of Naval Research

OSHA – Occupational Safety and Health Administration
OSTP – Office of Science and Technology Policy
OTA – Office of Technology Assessment
OTIR – Office of Technology and Industrial Relations

PA – Program Announcement
PDB – Protein Data Bank
PFGRC – Pathogen Functional Genomics Resource Center
PSAC – Presidents Science Advisory Committee
PSI – Protein Structure Initiative

RAID – Rapid Access to Intervention Development
RFA – Request for Applications
RTLA – Reach Through License Agreements

SBIR – Small Business Innovation Research
SDI – Strategic Defense Initiative
SEP – Special Emphasis Panels
SNP – Single Nucleotide Polymorphisms
SPORE – Specialized Programs of Research Excellence
SSC – Superconducting Super Collider
STC – Science and Technology Centers
STTR – Small Business Technology Transfer

TIGR – The Institute for Genomic Research

UIP – Unconventional Innovations Program
URA – Universities Research Association
USDA – United States Department of Agriculture

VA – Department of Veterans Affairs
VRC – Vaccine Research Center

WHI – Women's Health Initiative

Contents

Executive Summary

The nature of biomedical research has been evolving in recent years. Relatively small projects initiated by single investigators have traditionally been and continue to be the mainstay of cancer research, as well as biomedical research in other fields. Recently, however, technological advances that make it easier to study the vast complexity of biological systems have led to the initiation of projects with a larger scale and scope (Figure ES-1). For instance, a new approach to biological experimentation known as "discovery science" first aims to develop a detailed inventory of genes, proteins, and metabolites in a particular cell type or tissue as a key information source. But even that information is not sufficient to understand the cell's complexity, so the ultimate goal of such research is to identify and characterize the elaborate networks of gene and protein interactions in the entire system that contribute to disease. This concept of systems biology is based on the premise that a disease can be fully comprehended only when its cause is understood from the molecular to the organismal level. For example, rather than focusing on single aberrant genes or pathways, it is essential to understand the comprehensive and complex nature of cancer cells and their interaction with surrounding tissues. In many cases, large-scale analyses in which many parameters can be studied at once may be the most efficient and effective way to extract functional information and interactions from such complex biological systems.

The Human Genome Project is the biggest and best-known large-scale biomedical research project undertaken to date. Another project of that size is not likely to be launched in the near future, but many other

Conventional small-scale research $\rightarrow$ **Large-scale** $\rightarrow$ **Very large-scale collaborative research**

Smaller, more specific goals	$\rightarrow$	Broad goals (encompassing an entire field of inquiry)
Short-term objectives	$\rightarrow$	Requires long-range strategic planning
Relatively shorter time frame	$\rightarrow$	Often a longer time frame
Lower total cost, higher unit cost	$\rightarrow$	Higher total cost, lower unit cost
Hypothesis driven, undefined deliverables	$\rightarrow$	Problem-directed with well-defined deliverables and endpoints
Small peer review group approval sufficient	$\rightarrow$	Acceptance by the field as a whole important
Minimal management structure	$\rightarrow$	Larger, more complex management structure
Minimal oversight by funders	$\rightarrow$	More oversight by funders
Single principal investigator	$\rightarrow$	Multi-investigator and multi-institutional
More dependent on scientists in training	$\rightarrow$	More dependent on technical staff
Generally funded by unsolicited, investigator-initiated (R01) grants	$\rightarrow$	Often funded through solicited cooperative agreements
More discipline-oriented	$\rightarrow$	Often interdisciplinary
Takes advantage of infrastructure and technologies generated by large-scale projects	$\rightarrow$	Develops scientific research capacity, infrastructure, and technologies
May or may not involve bioinformatics	$\rightarrow$	Data and outcome analysis highly dependent on bioinformatics

FIGURE ES-1   The range of attributes that may characterize scientific research. There is no absolute distinction—indeed there is much overlap—between the characteristic of small- and large-scale research. Rather, these characteristics vary along a continuum that extends from traditional independent small-scale projects through very large, collaborative projects. Any single project may share some characteristics with either of these extremes.

projects that fall somewhere between the Human Genome Project and the traditional small projects have already been initiated, and many more have been contemplated. Indeed, the director of the National Institutes of Health (NIH) recently presented to his advisory council a "road map" for the agency's future that includes a greater emphasis on "revolutionary methods of research" focused on scientific questions too complex to be addressed by the single-investigator scientific approach. He noted that the NIH grant process will need to be adapted to accommodate this new large-scale approach to scientific investigation, which may conflict with traditional paradigms for proposing, funding, and managing science projects that were designed for smaller-scale, hypothesis-driven research.

The recent interest in adopting large-scale research methods has generated many questions, then, as to how such research in the biomedical sciences should be financed and conducted. Accordingly, the National Cancer Policy Board determined that a careful examination of these issues was warranted at this time. The purpose of this study was to (1) define the concept of "large-scale science" with respect to cancer research; (2) identify examples of ongoing large-scale projects to determine the current state of the field; (3) identify obstacles to the implementation of large-scale projects in biomedical research; and (4) make recommendations for improving the process for conducting large-scale biomedical science projects, should such projects be undertaken in the future.

Although the initial intent of this study was to examine large-scale cancer research, it quickly became clear that issues pertaining to large-scale science projects have broad implications that cut across all sectors and fields of biomedical research. Large-scale endeavors in the biomedical sciences often involve multiple disciplines and contribute to many fields and specialties. The Human Genome Project is a classic example of this concept, in that its products can benefit all fields of biology and biomedicine. The same is likely to be true for many other large-scale projects now under consideration or underway, such as the Protein Structure Initiative (PSI) and the International HapMap Project. Furthermore, given the funding structures of NIH, the launch of a large-scale project in one field could potentially impact progress as well as funding in other fields. Thus, while this report emphasizes examples from cancer research whenever feasible, the committee's recommendations are generally not specific to the National Cancer Institute (NCI) or to the field of cancer research; rather, they are directed toward the biomedical research community as a whole. Indeed, it is the committee's belief that all fields of biomedical research, including cancer research, could benefit from implementation of the recommendations presented herein.

Ideally, large-scale and small-scale research should complement each other and work synergistically to advance the field of biomedical research in the long term. For example, many large-scale projects generate hypotheses that can then be tested in smaller research projects. However, the new large-scale research opportunities are challenging traditional academic research structures because the projects are bigger, more costly, often more technologically sophisticated, and require greater planning and oversight. These challenges raise the question of how the large-scale approach to biomedical research could be improved if such projects are to be undertaken in the future. The committee concluded that such improvement could be achieved by adopting the seven recommendations presented here to address these issues.

The first three recommendations suggest a number of changes in the way scientific opportunities for large-scale research are initially assessed as they emerge from the scientific community, as well as in the way specific projects are subsequently selected, funded, launched, and evaluated (Table ES-1). Although the procedures of NIH and other federal agencies have a degree of flexibility that has allowed some large-scale research endeavors to be undertaken, a mechanism is needed through which input from innovators in research can be routinely collected and incorporated into the institutional decisionmaking processes. Also needed is a more standard mechanism for vetting various proposals for large-scale projects. For example, none of the large projects initiated by NCI to date has been evaluated in a systematic manner. There is also a need for greater planning and oversight by federal sponsors during both the initiation and phase-out of a large-scale project. Careful assessment of past and current large-scale projects to identify best practices and determine whether the large-scale approach adds value to the traditional models of research would also provide highly useful information for future endeavors.

> **Recommendation 1: NIH and other federal funding agencies that support large-scale biomedical science (including the National Science Foundation [NSF], the U.S. Department of Energy [DOE], the U.S. Department of Agriculture [USDA], and the U.S. Department of Defense [DOD]) should develop a more open and systematic method for assessing important new research opportunities emerging from the scientific community in which a large-scale approach is likely to achieve the scientific goals more effectively or efficiently than traditional research efforts.**

- This method should include a mechanism for soliciting and evaluating proposals from individuals or small groups as well as from large groups, but in either case, broad consultation within the relevant scientific community should occur before funding is made available, perhaps through ad hoc public conferences. Whenever feasible, these discussions should be NIH-wide and multidisciplinary.
- An NIH-wide, trans-institute panel of experts appointed by the NIH director would facilitate the vetting process for assessing scientific opportunities that could benefit from a large-scale approach.
- Once the most promising concepts for large-scale research have been selected by the director's panel, appropriate guidelines for peer review of specific project proposals should be established. These guidelines should be applied by the institutions that oversee the projects.

TABLE ES-1 Summary of the Challenges Associated with Large-Scale Biomedical Research Projects, and the Committee's Recommendations to Overcome These Difficulties

Difficulties Associated with Large-Scale Projects	Potential Paths to Solutions
No systematic method for assessing large-scale biomedical research opportunities exists.	Develop an NIH-wide mechanism for soliciting and reviewing proposals for large-scale projects, with input from all relevant sectors of biomedical science.
Carefully planning and orchestrating the launch as well as the phase out of a large-scale project is difficult, but imperative for its long term success and efficiency.	Clear but flexible plans for entry into and phase out from projects should be developed before funding is provided.
There are very few precedents to guide the planning and oversight of large-scale endeavors in biomedical science.	NCI and NIH should commission a thorough analysis of their recent large-scale initiatives to determine whether those efforts have been effective and efficient in meeting their stated goals and to aid in the planning of future large-scale projects.
It is difficult to recruit and retain qualified scientific managers and staff for large-scale projects.	Institutions should develop new ways to recognize and reward scientific collaborations and team-building efforts.
It can be costly and difficult for investigators to maintain reagents produced through large-scale projects and to share them with the research community.	NIH should provide funding to preserve and distribute reagents and other research tools once they have been created.
Licensing strategies can affect the availability of research tools produced by and used for large-scale research projects.	NIH should examine systematically the impact of licensing strategies and should promote licensing practices that facilitate broad access to research tools.
A seamless transition between discovery and clinical application is lacking.	Consideration should be given to pursuing projects initiated by academic scientists in cooperation with industry to achieve large-scale research goals.

- Collaborations among institutes could encourage participation by smaller institutes that may not have the resources to launch their own large-scale projects.
- NIH should continue to explore alternative funding mechanisms for large-scale endeavors, perhaps including approaches similar to those used by NCI's Unconventional Innovations Program, as well as funding collaborations with industry and other federal funding agencies.

- International collaborations should be encouraged, but an approach for achieving such cooperation should be determined on a case by case basis.

Recommendation 2: Large-scale research endeavors should have clear but flexible plans for entry into and phase out from projects once the stated ends have been achieved.

- It is essential to define the goals of a project clearly and to monitor and assess its progress regularly against well-defined milestones.
- Carefully planning and orchestrating the launch of a large-scale project is imperative for its long-term success and efficiency.
- NIH should be very cautious about establishing permanent infrastructures, such as centers or institutes, to undertake large-scale projects, in order to avoid the accumulation of additional Institutes via this mechanism.
- Historically, NIH has not had a good mechanism for phasing out established research programs, but large-scale projects should not become institutionalized by default simply because of their size.
- If national centers with short-term missions are to be established, this should be done with a clear understanding that they are temporary and are not meant to continue once a project has been completed.
  - Leasing space is one way to facilitate downsizing upon completion of a project.
  - Phase-out funding could enable investigators to downsize over a period of 2–3 years.

Recommendation 3: NCI and NIH, as well as other federal funding agencies that support large-scale biomedical science, should commission a thorough analysis of their recent large-scale initiatives once they are well established to determine whether those efforts have been effective and efficient in achieving their stated goals and to aid in the planning of future large-scale projects.

- NIH should develop a set of metrics for assessing the technical and scientific output (such as data and research tools) of large-scale projects. The assessment should include an evaluation of whether the field has benefited from such a project in terms of increased speed of discoveries and their application or a reduction in costs.
- The assessment should be undertaken by external, independent peer review panels with relevant expertise that include academic, government, and industry scientists.
- To help guide future large-scale projects, the assessment should pay particular attention to a project's management and organiza-

tional structure, including how scientific and program managers and staff were selected, trained, and retained and how well they performed.

- The assessment should include tracking of any trainees involved in a project (graduate students and postdoctoral scientists) to determine the value of the training environment and the impact on career trajectories.
- The assessment should examine the impact of industry contracts or collaborations within large-scale research projects. Industry has many potential strengths to offer such projects, including efficiency and effective project management and staffing, but intellectual property issues represent a potential barrier to such collaborations. Thus, some balance must be sought between providing incentives for producing the data and facilitating the research community's access to the resultant data.
  - In pursuing large-scale projects with industry, NIH should carefully consider the data dissemination goals of the endeavor before making the funds available.
  - To the extent appropriate, NIH should mandate timely and unrestricted release of data within the terms of the grant or contract, in the same spirit as the Bermuda rules adopted for the release of data in the Human Genome Project.

The committee has formulated four additional recommendations aimed at improving the conduct of possible future large-scale projects. These recommendations emerged from the committee's identification of various potential obstacles to conducting a large-scale research project successfully and efficiently. To begin with, human resources are key to the success of any large-scale project. If large-scale projects are deemed worthy of substantial sums of federal support, they also clearly warrant the highest-caliber staff to perform and oversee the work. But if qualified individuals, especially at the doctoral level, are expected to participate in such undertakings, they must have sufficient incentives to take on the risks and responsibilities involved. In particular, effective administrative management and committed scientific leadership are crucial for meeting expected milestones on schedule and within budget; thus the success of a large-scale project is greatly dependent upon the skills and knowledge of the scientists and administrators who manage it, including those within the federal funding agencies. However, it may be quite difficult to recruit staff with the skills to meet this need because of the unusual status of such managerial positions within the scientific career structure, and because scientists rarely undergo formal training in management. Young investigators and trainees also need recognition for their efforts that contribute to elaborate, long-term, and large multi-institutional efforts. Thus, the committee concluded that both universities and government agencies need to develop new approaches for assessing teamwork and management, as well as novel ways of recognizing and rewarding accomplishment in such positions.

Recommendation 4: Institutions should develop the necessary incentives for recruiting and retaining qualified scientific managers and staff for large-scale projects, and for recognizing and rewarding scientific collaborations and team-building efforts.

- Funding agencies should develop appropriate career paths for individuals who serve as program managers for the large-scale projects they fund.
- Academic institutions should develop appropriate career paths, including suitable criteria for performance evaluation and promotion, for those individuals who manage and staff large-scale collaborative projects carried out under their purview.
- Industry and The National Laboratories may both serve as instructive models in achieving these goals, as they have a history of rewarding scientists for their participation in team-oriented research.
- It is important to establish guiding principles for such issues as equitable pay and benefits, job stability, and potential for advancement to avoid relegating these valuable scientists and managers to a "second-tier" status. Federal agencies should provide adequate funding to universities engaged in large-scale biomedical research projects so that these individuals can be sufficiently compensated for their role and contribution.
- Universities, especially those engaged in large-scale research, should develop training programs for scientists involved in such projects. Examples include courses dealing with such topics as managing teams of people and working toward milestones within timelines. Input from industry experts who deal routinely with these issues would be highly valuable.

The committee also identified potential impediments to deriving the greatest benefits from the products of large-scale endeavors in terms of scientific progress for biomedical research in general. Large-scale projects are most likely to speed the progress of biomedical research as a whole when their products are made widely available to the broad scientific community. However, concerns have been raised in recent years about the willingness and ability of scientists and their institutions to share data, reagents, and other tools derived from their research. Since a primary goal of many large-scale biomedical research projects is to produce data and research tools, NIH should facilitate the sharing of data and the distribution of reagents to the extent feasible. Currently, NIH grants generally do not provide funds for this purpose, making it difficult for investigators to maintain reagents and share them with the research community. This obstacle could be reduced if NIH provided such funds for large-scale research projects.

> **Recommendation 5: NIH should draft contracts with industry to preserve reagents and other research tools and distribute them to the scientific community once they have been produced through large-scale projects.**
>
> - The Pathogen Functional Genomics Resource Center, established through a contract with the National Institute of Allergy and Infectious Diseases, could serve as a model for this undertaking.
> - The distribution of standardized and quality-controlled reagents and tools would improve the quality of the data obtained through research and make it easier to compare data from different investigators.
> - Producing the reagents and making them widely available to many researchers would be more cost-effective than providing funds to a few scientists to produce their own.

An issue closely related to the sharing of data and reagents is the licensing of intellectual property. Many concerns have been raised in recent years about the challenges and expenses associated with the transfer of patented technology from one organization to another. Innovations that can be used as research tools may offer the greatest challenge in this regard because it is difficult to predict the future applications and value of a particular tool, and because a number of different tools may be needed for a single research project. Since many large-scale projects in the biosciences aim to produce data and other tools for future research, this subject is especially salient for large-scale research. The committee concluded that NIH should continue to promote the broad accessibility of research tools derived from federally funded large-scale research to the extent feasible, while at the same time considering the appropriate role for intellectual property rights in a given project. However, in the absence of adequate information and scholarly assessment, it is difficult to determine how NIH could best accomplish that goal. Thus, the committee recommends that such an assessment be undertaken, and that appropriate actions be taken based on the findings of the study.

> **Recommendation 6: NIH should commission a study to examine systematically the ways in which licensing practices affect the avail-**

ability of research tools produced by and used for large-scale biomedical research projects.

- Whenever possible, NIH and NCI should use their leverage and resources to promote the free and open exchange of scientific knowledge and information, and to help minimize the time and expense of technology transfer.
- Depending on the findings of the proposed study, NIH should promote licensing practices that facilitate broad access to research tools by issuing licensing guidelines for NIH-funded discoveries.

In addition to the role of federal funding agencies, the committee considered the role of industry and philanthropies in conducting large-scale biomedical research. Public–private collaborations provide a way to share the costs and risks of innovative research, as well as the benefits. Philanthropies and other nonprofit organizations can play an important role in launching nontraditional projects that do not fit well with federal funding mechanisms. Pharmaceutical and biotechnology companies also make enormous contributions to biomedical research worldwide. Traditionally, the role of independent companies has been to pursue applied research aimed at producing an end product; however, the distinction between "applied" and "basic" research has blurred in recent years, in part because of novel approaches used for drug discovery and development. A recent focus by academic scientists on translational research, which aims to translate fundamental discoveries into clinically useful practices, has further obscured the distinction.

Several recent projects initiated and funded by industry or carried out in cooperation with industry and nonprofit organizations clearly demonstrate the potential value of contributions by these entities to large-scale research endeavors. The Single Nucleotide Polymorphism, or SNP, consortium is a prime example of how effective these sectors can be when involved in a large-scale research projects. Industry in particular has many inherent strengths that could be brought to bear on large-scale biomedical research efforts, such as experience in coordinating and managing teams of scientists working toward a common goal. Combining the respective strengths of academia and industry could optimize the pace of biomedical research and development, potentially leading to more rapid improvements in human health. Thus, the committee recommends that cooperation between academia and industry be encouraged for large-scale research projects whenever feasible.

Recommendation 7: Given the changing nature of biomedical research, consideration should be given to pursuing projects initiated by academic scientists in cooperation with industry to achieve the

goals of large-scale research. When feasible, such cooperative efforts could entail collaborative projects, as well as direct funding of academic research by industry, if the goals of the research are mutually beneficial.

- Academia is generally best suited for making scientific discoveries, while the strength of industry most often lies in its ability to develop or add value to these discoveries.
- Establishing a more seamless connection between the two endeavors could greatly facilitate translational research and thus speed clinical applications of new discoveries.

Great strides in biomedical research have been made in recent decades, due largely to a robust investigator-initiated research enterprise. Recent technological advances have provided new opportunities to further accelerate the pace of discovery through large-scale research initiatives that can provide valuable information and tools to facilitate this traditional approach to experimentation. Recent large-scale collaborations have also allowed scientists to tackle complex research questions that could not readily be addressed by a single investigator or institution. The current leadership of NIH and many scientists in the field clearly have expressed an interest in integrating the discovery approach to biomedical science with hypothesis-driven experimentation. As a result, at least some large-scale endeavors in the biomedical sciences are likely to be undertaken in the future as well. But because the large-scale approach is relatively new to the life sciences, there are few precedents to follow or learn from when planning and launching a new large-scale project. Moreover, there has been little formal or scholarly assessment of large-scale projects already undertaken.

Now is the time to address the critical issues identified in this report in order to optimize future investments in large-scale endeavors, whatever they may be. The ultimate goal of biomedical research, both large- and small-scale, is to advance knowledge and provide society with useful innovations. Determining the best and most efficient method for accomplishing that goal, however, is a continuing and evolving challenge. Following the recommendations presented here could facilitate a move toward a more open, inclusive, and accountable approach to large-scale biomedical research, and help strike the appropriate balance between large- and small-scale research to maximize progress in understanding and controlling human disease.

1

Introduction

Historically, most cancer research has been conducted through small independent projects initiated by individual investigators with relatively small research groups. Such research is driven by focused hypotheses addressing specific biological questions. There will always be a need for this traditional approach to research; in recent years, however, it has also become more feasible to undertake projects on a broader and larger scale, thereby developing extensive pools of data and research tools that can facilitate those more conventional efforts. Large-scale science projects, in which many investigators often work toward a common goal, have become quite common, and perhaps even the norm in some fields of scientific research, such as high-energy physics (Galison and Hevly, 1992; Heilbron and Kevles, 1988). The large-scale approach has also been used for decades or even centuries to develop astronomical charts and geological and oceanic maps that can be used as tools for scientific inquiry (see Appendix). However, the concept is still relatively new in the biomedical sciences, including cancer research.

This new paradigm of biomedical research has become possible in part through technological advances that allow for high-throughput data collection and analysis—an approach referred to as "discovery science." Traditional biomedical research is conducted by small groups that test hypotheses and are interactive but not highly collaborative, whereas large-scale biology often involves large, highly collaborative groups that deal with the high-throughput collection and analysis of large bodies of data. The two approaches can be synergistic in the long term when large-scale projects produce data that can be used to generate hypotheses, which can then be tested with smaller-scale experiments.

The biggest and most visible large-scale research project conducted in biology to date is the Human Genome Project (HGP), aimed at mapping and sequencing the human genome. While not exclusive to the study of cancer, the products of this project can serve as research tools for the study of cancer, and thus will have a far-reaching influence on the progress and direction of cancer research in the future. As a result, there is considerable interest in the field of cancer research in developing other similar projects with broad potential benefits. Projects of the scope and scale of the HGP are perhaps unlikely to be launched in the foreseeable future, but many projects that are larger or broader in scope than traditional efforts are already under way. One such initiative in cancer research is the Cancer Genome Anatomy Project (CGAP) of the National Cancer Institute.[1] The goal of this project is to develop gene expression profiles of normal, precancerous, and cancerous cells, which could then be used by many investigators to search for new methods of cancer detection, diagnosis, and treatment.

At the same time, this recent interest in large-scale biomedical science projects raises many questions regarding how such projects should be evaluated, funded, initiated, organized, managed, and staffed. Once it has been decided that a large-scale approach is appropriate for achieving a specific goal, a variety of issues—such as staffing and scientific training; challenges in communication, data sharing, and decision making; and intellectual property issues (patenting, licensing, and trade secrets)—must be considered in choosing the appropriate venue for the research. Difficulties can also arise because research within large-scale projects may be conducted by multiple institutions and is often multidisciplinary, thus requiring management of diverse complementary components. In addition, such projects often require strategic planning with clearly defined endpoints and deliverables, they often entail technology development, and they generally have longer timeframes than conventional research. These characteristics may not mesh well with the traditional organization and operation of research institutions, especially with respect to funding mechanisms and peer review, ownership of intellectual property, scientific training, career advancement, and planning and management oversight within academic institutions.

Many decisions must be made before a large-scale project is launched, such as where the funding will come from and how it will be made available to investigators; what projects and institutions will be funded; and how activities will be organized, managed, completed, and evaluated.

---

[1] See <http://cgap.nci.nih.gov/>.

The National Institutes of Health (NIH), in contrast to some other federal agencies, has not developed a standardized or institutionalized approach for making decisions about large-scale science projects, which require a long-term funding commitment. For very large projects that involve multiple federal agencies, there is also a need to coordinate funding. Moreover, such projects often attract international cooperation, so mechanisms for addressing such cooperation need to be in place. Finally, because large-scale science is very expensive, there is always concern that it will reduce the pool of money available for smaller, traditionally funded projects and thereby slow the progress of innovation. As noted above, however, there should ideally be a long-term synergy between large- and small-scale projects in biomedical science, with the former providing new research tools and resources for the advancement of the latter.

A variety of models exist for carrying out large-scale biological research projects, and each has its strengths and advantages. As noted earlier, the Human Genome Project is the largest and most visible undertaking in biology to date. In the United States, public funding for the project came from both NIH and the U.S. Department of Energy (DOE), but only after considerable debate over the merit of the project, the best way to accomplish its goals, and how to fund it adequately without reducing support for other aspects of biomedical research. In the end, significant investment was also made by private industry. With the successful completion of the draft sequence (Lander et al., 2001; Venter et al., 2001), the project is now being hailed as a remarkable example of what can be accomplished through a large-scale science venture in biology. But is this the best or only way to take on future large-scale biomedical research? There are other strategies for funding and organizing such projects, some of which have never been used in biology but have worked well in other scientific fields.

Because the concept of large-scale science is relatively new to the field of biomedical research, and there is increasing interest is using this research format to advance the study of cancer, the National Cancer Policy Board determined that it would be useful at this time to address some of the issues and questions outlined above. The purpose of the study documented in this report, then, was to:

- Define the concept of large-scale biomedical science, with a particular focus on its application to cancer research.
- Examine the current state of large-scale science in biomedical research (what is being done and how).
- Examine other potential models of large-scale biomedical research.

The National Cancer Policy Board

The National Cancer Policy Board was established in 1997 within the Institute of Medicine and the National Research Council to address broad policy issues that affect cancer research and care in the United States, and to recommend ways of advancing the nation's effort to combat the disease. The board, consisting of members drawn from outside the federal government, includes health care consumers, providers, and researchers in a variety of disciplines in the sciences and humanities.

The board meets at least three times per year to review progress; discuss emerging issues; and gather information and views from representatives of the private and public sectors, including many federal and state agencies that sponsor or conduct related work. The board analyzes information; issues reports and recommendations, prepared under its direction by professional staff members; and may commission papers and hold workshops in support of those projects. It also oversees reports prepared by committees appointed to conduct a specific task.

- Examine the ways in which the field of biomedical research is adapting to the inclusion of large-scale projects.
- Identify obstacles to the implementation of large-scale projects in cancer research.
- Provide policy recommendations for improving the process for conducting large-scale projects in cancer research should they be undertaken in the future.

This report is organized as follows.

Chapter 2 develops a working definition of "large-scale biomedical research" within the framework of this report. It also provides brief examples of the types of projects that may be amenable to the large-scale research approach, as well as a brief overview of the challenges and impediments involved in using this approach.

Chapter 3 provides in-depth information about a wide variety of past and current large-scale research models or strategies undertaken by the National Cancer Institute (NCI) and other branches of NIH, as well as examples from outside of NIH, including both public and private endeavors.

Chapter 4 presents an overview of the available funding sources and mechanisms for scientific research, with emphasis on how they are adapting to the emergence of large-scale projects in the biomedical sciences.

Chapter 5 reviews the role of project management, oversight, and assessment in large-scale research endeavors.

Chapter 6 provides a general overview of trends in the training and career development of biomedical scientists, and includes a discussion of how large-scale projects may influence or be affected by these trends.

Chapter 7 examines the role of intellectual property in biomedical research, with particular emphasis on the availability of large-scale data and research tools.

Chapter 8 summarizes the key findings of the study and presents the committee's recommendations.

2

Defining "Large-Scale Science" in Biomedical Research

The term "large-scale science" is defined and used in many different ways (National Research Council, 1994). The concept can vary greatly across fields and disciplines, or even across funding agencies; what is "large" for biology, for example, may be quite modest for space science or high-energy physics. Similarly, a large project in cancer research may pale in comparison with the Human Genome Project. The concept may also vary over time, in part as a result of technological advances. For instance, because of enormous advances in DNA sequencing technology, the time and cost of sequencing a mammalian genome are now considerably lower than was the case when the Human Genome Project (HGP) was launched; thus such projects are becoming less likely to be viewed as exceptional, large-scale undertakings.

Unfortunately, the concepts of "large" and "small" science are often stereotyped in discussions of relative merit. Yet inaccurate generalizations belie the complexity of the terms. It is therefore essential to define clearly what is and is not meant by large-scale science within the context of this study. For the purposes of this report, a project may be characterized as large-scale if it serves any or all of the following three objectives:

- Creation of large-scale products (e.g., generating masses of related data to accomplish a single broad mission or goal)
- Developing large-scale infrastructure (e.g., generating databases and bioinformatics tools, or advancing the speed and volume of research through improved instrumentation)

• Addressing large and complex but focused problems that have a broad impact on biomedical or cancer research and may require interactions or collaborations among multiple investigators and institutions

Biomedical research projects are not easily classified as either small- or large-scale because there is considerable overlap among the attributes that could be used to define them. Each attribute can be characterized along a continuum from what is typical for conventional small-scale research to what is typical for a very large-scale, collaborative endeavor (see Figure 2-1). Any given project may have a combination of attributes that fall on different points along this continuum. Large-scale projects tend to be very resource intensive (where the term "resource" may include

Conventional small-scale research → Large-scale → Very large-scale collaborative research

Smaller, more specific goals	→	Broad goals (encompassing an entire field of inquiry)
Short-term objectives	→	Requires long-range strategic planning
Relatively shorter time frame	→	Often a longer time frame
Lower total cost, higher unit cost	→	Higher total cost, lower unit cost
Hypothesis driven, undefined deliverables	→	Problem-directed with well-defined deliverables and endpoints
Small peer review group approval sufficient	→	Acceptance by the field as a whole important
Minimal management structure	→	Larger, more complex management structure
Minimal oversight by funders	→	More oversight by funders
Single principal investigator	→	Multi-investigator and multi-institutional
More dependent on scientists in training	→	More dependent on technical staff
Generally funded by unsolicited, investigator-initiated (R01) grants	→	Often funded through solicited cooperative agreements
More discipline-oriented	→	Often interdisciplinary
Takes advantage of infrastructure and technologies generated by large-scale projects	→	Develops scientific research capacity, infrastructure, and technologies
May or may not involve bioinformatics	→	Data and outcome analysis highly dependent on bioinformatics

FIGURE 2-1 The range of attributes that may characterize scientific research. There is no absolute distinction—indeed there is much overlap—between the characteristic of small- and large-scale research. Rather, these characteristics vary along a continuum that extends from traditional independent small-scale projects through very large, collaborative projects. Any single project may share some characteristics with either of these extremes.

money, space and equipment, and personnel); thus they require collective agreement or buy-in from the larger scientific community, rather than just a small number of experts in a subspecialty. To achieve such agreement, large-scale projects must be mission or goal oriented, with clearly defined endpoints and deliverables that create infrastructure or scientific capacity to enhance future research endeavors. Such infrastructure may include products such as databases and new technologies that could be used as research tools by a significant portion of the scientific community and would provide a common platform for research. In other words, a major intent of such projects is to enable the progress of smaller projects. Technological advances have created a need for data-rich foundations for many cutting-edge research proposals that are investigator initiated and hypothesis driven. Thus, many large-scale projects can be thought of as inductive or generating hypotheses, as opposed to deductive or testing hypotheses, the latter being more commonly the realm of smaller-scale research. Large-scale collaborative projects may also complement smaller projects by achieving an important, complex goal that could not be accomplished through the traditional model of single-investigator, small-scale research. In either case, the objective of a large-scale project should be to produce a public good—an end product that is valuable for society and is useful to many or all investigators in the field.

Unlike traditional investigator-initiated projects, research within large-scale projects may be conducted by many investigators at multiple institutions or sometimes even in numerous countries. Such research is also often multidisciplinary in nature. Thus, the work may require external coordination and management of various complementary components. It can also be very challenging to analyze the resultant masses of data and to evaluate the outcomes and scientific capacity of such collaborative research. Furthermore, these unconventional projects have larger budgets than most projects undertaken in the biomedical sciences, so it can be difficult to launch them using the traditional NIH funding mechanisms. In principle, however, the unit cost of collecting data in a large-scale project should be lower. These projects also often have a longer time frame than smaller projects, and thus require more strategic planning with intermediate goals and endpoints, as well as a phase-out strategy.

Within the context of this report, the definition of large-scale biomedical science does not include exceptionally large laboratories that are headed by a single principal investigator who is simply funded by multiple grants obtained through conventional funding sources. Nor does it include traditional program (P0-1) grants, in which multiple investigators are provided funding for independent but somewhat related small-scale projects. Unlike some other fields, large-scale biomedical science usually does not entail very large research facilities, such as the Fermi National

Accelerator Laboratory for research in high-energy physics. In addition, large-scale biomedical science is not defined by whether it is basic, translational, or clinical research, but could entail any of these categories. For example, cancer clinical cooperative groups may be seen as a form of clinical large-scale science. The NCI, unlike other NIH Institutes, has set aside a sum of money to support a large infrastructure to carry out clinical studies.

Ultimately, the distinction between small- and large-scale biomedical science is determined by the needs and difficulties entailed in achieving a given research goal, and by the current capabilities in a particular field. For example, many traditional investigator-initiated projects in biomedical research focus on improving our understanding of genes or proteins that are thought to be of biological interest. In contrast, unconventional large-scale projects take advantage of economies of scale to produce relatively standardized data on entire classes or categories of biological questions. Thus, as noted earlier, they may reveal novel areas of research for follow-up by smaller science projects, and they also provide essential tools and databases for subsequent research. Large-scale projects may be the most suitable approach for biological questions that can be addressed more effectively or efficiently by coordinating the work of many scientists to produce clearly defined deliverables through the development and use of advanced technology. Smaller projects are more suitable for addressing specific, hypothesis-driven scientific questions, which are essential for the steady progress and evolution of the field. Such projects are undertaken by many individual investigators, and often yield unexpected findings that can dramatically alter the course of future research.

Ideally, as noted in Chapter 1, there should be a synergism between large- and small-scale science in the long term. For example, one of the frequently cited benefits of the Human Genome Project (HGP) is that it could facilitate faster, less costly, and easier location and identification of genes that promote disease when mutated—a goal of many smaller conventional science projects. Both large and small science endeavors can make important contributions to a particular field, and the appropriate balance between the two may vary over time. Moreover, because biomedical research in general is becoming increasingly interdisciplinary and technology driven, there may be greater opportunities to reap the benefits of large-scale projects.

EXAMPLES OF POTENTIAL LARGE-SCALE BIOMEDICAL RESEARCH PROJECTS

Although the number and variety of potential large-scale biomedical research projects are probably limitless, there are several areas that have been widely discussed and may be more feasible now or in the near future. In fact, a number of such projects are already under way with support from a variety of sources, including industry, government, and nonprofit organizations. Several examples of potential projects in four areas—genomics, structural biology and proteomics, bioinformatics, and diagnostics and biomarker research—are discussed briefly here as a means of elaborating on the working definition of large-scale biomedical science used for this report. Some of these examples are discussed in greater detail in Chapter 3 as models for conducting large-scale bioscience research.

Large-scale biomedical research differs from many large-scale undertakings in the physical sciences in the sense that partial completion or partial success of a project to collect large pools of biological data would still be useful. As a result, it may be less risky to undertake a long-range, large-scale project in the biosciences when future budgets are in question. For example, production of a partial rather than a comprehensive catalog of protein structures could still be quite useful to the scientific community. In contrast, the building of a large-scale facility, such as a superconducting super collider or the Fermi Laboratory is useful only if the facility were completed and then used successfully by members of the scientific community to generate data. Likewise, the Manhattan Project to develop the atomic bomb would have been deemed a failure if only partial progress had been made in attaining the ultimate goal.

Genomics

Thousands of people are now working in genomics—a field that did not exist 15 years ago. (For a recent summary of genomics funding, see Figure 4-3 in Chapter 4). The completion of the draft sequence of the human genome is a tremendous achievement, but a great deal of additional work is needed to realize the full value of this accomplishment. DNA sequences provide only limited information about a species. Many additional layers of information, regulation, and interaction must be deciphered if we are to truly understand the workings of the human body in health and disease. Of the many types of biological information, DNA sequences are among the easiest to obtain but the most difficult to interpret—that is, they provide minimal information regarding structure and function. Thus, the sequence of the human genome in itself does not reveal the "secret of life," but it is an important tool for answering many questions in biomedical research.

For example, defining and characterizing the many regulatory elements in DNA will improve our understanding of how, when, and why various gene products are generated in both health and disease. The availability of genome databases should facilitate the development of "whole genome" screens that can be used to assess the expression of all genes in a given sample or to examine the resulting phenotypes when the genome is systematically altered to over- or underexpress the genes. There is also great interest in defining variation among humans with regard to genetic polymorphisms in disease-related genes and disease modifier genes—small differences in the DNA sequence of individuals that may not be directly responsible for disease per se, but may lead to subtle differences in susceptibility for various diseases, including cancer, or may contribute to the variability in response to therapies. Polymorphisms can also serve as markers for locating genes that do directly contribute to disease when mutated.

Other examples of genomics-related projects include generating databases of full-length cDNAs—DNA sequences that are complementary to messenger RNAs, which actually code for proteins, and thus have intervening "intron" sequences removed. These resources could then be used as tools to study gene expression and function. This is one of the aims of NCI's Cancer Genome Anatomy Project (CGAP). There is also great interest in sequencing the genomes of organisms that serve as experimental or comparative models for biomedical research.

Structural Biology and Proteomics

Structural biology is the study of protein composition and configuration (Burley, 2000). The term "proteomics" refers to the study of the structure and function of the "proteome"—that is, all proteins produced by the genome. The expressed products of a given genome can vary greatly across cell and tissue types, and over time, within the same cell. There are many opportunities for biochemical modification, regulation, and translocation between the time when transcription of the DNA into RNA is initiated and when the final protein product is removed or eliminated from the cells. Furthermore, proteins do not work alone, but within multisubunit structures and complex networks; thus there is an immensely sophisticated combinatorial complexity to deal with in trying to understand cellular or organismal function. The pathobiology of disease adds further layers of complexity that can be quite species-specific. In the case of cancer, for example, a great variety of mutations can be found that affect the structure, interactions, and function of proteins that play key roles in the regulation of cell growth and survival. Furthermore, the specific mutations present can vary greatly across different types of cancer, among individual patients, and even within different tissue layers and cells of a single tumor.

Analogies have been drawn between the HGP and the study of proteomics, but one major difference is the lack of a single objective with a clear endpoint. In the case of the HGP, the goal was simply to obtain a reference sequence for each of the chromosomes in a human cell. Because there is no single "human proteome," the endpoint will vary depending on what question is being addressed. In the case of cancer, for example, there could be great value in cataloging and studying the unique proteomes of cancer cells. Novel forms of proteins, altered interactions among proteins, and altered responses to normal regulation may be discovered.

Bioinformatics

In many aspects, biology is becoming an information science: many important questions in biology are now being addressed, at least in part, through interactions with computer science and applied mathematics. Scientists can now produce immense datasets that allow them to look at biological information in ways never before possible. For example, it is now theoretically possible to study complex and dynamic biological systems quantitatively (Lake and Hood, 2001). Once a large resource of biological data or information becomes available, however, it becomes a challenge to use that resource effectively. The new field of bioinformatics aims to develop the computational tools and protocols needed for establishing, maintaining, using, and analyzing large sets of data or biological information. Thus, bioinformatics may constitute one key component of a large-scale research project aimed at generating large datasets that encompass an entire field of inquiry. In cancer research, for example, it would be useful to catalog and characterize the key molecular changes cells undergo in the transition from a normal to a neoplastic and metastatic cell. The development of bioinformatics tools and resources could also potentially serve as a large-scale research project in itself, because the availability of standardized bioinformatics tools could lead to greater uniformity and use of data generated within smaller, more traditional science projects. There is a great need for a common language and platform for many applications.

Diagnostics and Biomarker Research

Much effort has been devoted to identifying and characterizing "molecular biomarkers" of cancer—any change at the biochemical or molecular level that may provide insight into how a particular cancer will behave, how it should be treated, and how it is responding to treatment. There is also great interest in using biomarkers for early detection, since some cancerous changes may be detectable by molecular methods before the cells have had a chance to grow into a tumor that can be detected by physical methods (usually imaging or palpation). For example, cancer cells can secrete abnormal proteins that might be detected by a blood test. Many potential markers have been studied over the years, but only a very few have proven to be clinically useful. However, recent advances in high-throughput technologies (such as those developed for genomics, proteomics, and bioinformatics) may make it easier to systematically search for and assess biomarker candidates.

Patient Databases and Specimen Banks

Collections of archived patient information—including clinical data, family history, and risk factors, as well as patient samples, such as tissue, blood, and urine—can be very useful for studying the genetics, biology, etiology, and epidemiology of diseases, especially when they are linked. Such collections of information can also be used to examine the long-term effects of medical interventions. Once established, these annotated data and specimen banks can be used to address new questions and hypotheses as they arise. Some of the challenges involved in developing this sort of research tool, in addition to the high cost, include concerns about scientists' access to the resource, as well as patient confidentiality and informed consent for future studies. Changing technology can also render older samples obsolete if the newer methods of analysis require a different method of sample preservation.

POTENTIAL OBSTACLES TO UNDERTAKING LARGE-SCALE BIOMEDICAL RESEARCH PROJECTS

Because large-scale science projects may not fit readily into the traditional molds for biomedical research, there are many factors to consider and obstacles to overcome in making decisions about whether and how to conduct such projects in cancer research. A brief overview of these topics is provided here to elaborate the working definition of large-scale science in cancer research. Each topic is covered in greater detail in Chapters 4 through 7.

Determining Appropriate Funding Mechanisms and Allocation of Funds

Buy-in by the leaders of the scientific community as a whole is important for the initiation of a large-scale research project, as this mode of operation is a relatively new concept in biology and has been met with resistance in the past. There should be some consensus that a large-scale approach to a scientific problem will add value, and will achieve a given goal more rapidly, more efficiently, or more completely than would be possible through conventional funding mechanisms. In other words, it should be clear that to forego a large-scale approach would result in a lost opportunity to achieve a certain goal, or significant delays and increased cost in the long run.

Once a large-scale science project has been agreed upon, funding sources must be identified. The number and variety of potential funding sources for biomedical research have increased greatly in the last 50 years. Sources include several government agencies, many private industries, and nonprofit organizations, each with a different culture, objectives, and traditions that may cause it to react quite differently to a given idea for a large-scale project. For example, industry can be expected to take a greater interest in projects that appear to offer potential near-term profits, whereas federal agencies are more likely to fund the generation of basic information that could be used as a research tool. However, these distinctions are rarely clear-cut in biology, and thus there is often overlapping interest and even competition among potential sponsors of large-scale research projects. In any case, the decision to offer funding and allocation of the funds are prerequisites for any large and complex project, as the traditional funding mechanisms in biomedical research were not designed for such endeavors.

Once funds have been designated for a large-scale biomedical research project, criteria must be established for determining which individuals, groups, or institutions will be awarded funds for specific components of the project. The vetting process for large-scale projects may require a different set of questions for evaluating the relative merits of applicants than those commonly raised for smaller projects. In some cases, more long-term planning than is typical of traditionally funded projects might be required to define the objectives, feasibility, and expected products of a large-scale project, including intermediate endpoints for measuring progress and assessing accountability. Such long-range planning is very challenging in a rapidly changing scientific field, and may be somewhat at odds with the nature of scientific exploration and discovery.

Organization and Management

There is no single formula for organizing and managing a large-scale research project. The approach can vary greatly depending on the goal and the methods chosen to achieve it. Nonetheless, it can be said that the organizational requirements of large-scale science projects are likely to be quite different from those of the more traditional academic approach to biomedical science. For large-scale projects, the work may need to be coordinated among multiple public and private research institutions, or across disciplines, funding agencies, and even national governments in the case of international projects.

The typical U.S. academic research laboratory is headed by a single principal investigator, who oversees the work of more-junior scientists—such as graduate students and postdoctoral fellows—as well as technicians. There tends to be relatively little hierarchical management of projects within such laboratories, and little or no management from external sources. Because the junior scientists are generally in training to become independent researchers, they should ideally spend much of their time learning techniques and developing their own independent lines of research.

Large-scale science projects, in contrast, often require external management and oversight to some degree so that the work of the participating groups can be coordinated and kept on track for meeting the program goals. Once a large-scale project has been launched, it is imperative to monitor and evaluate its progress against expected milestones, and to alter course if necessary. When a project requires a multidisciplinary approach, the potential problems of organization, management, and oversight are even greater because of difficulties in communicating across fields. This situation could make it more difficult to establish priorities and intermediate endpoints or milestones, which are essential for attaining the ultimate project goal. The ideal manager for external oversight would thus have extensive experience in all the relevant disciplines; however, such individuals may be rare because most current training programs tend to focus on a single discipline.

Because of these challenges, the industrial model of biomedical research may have much to offer large-scale research projects, even when they are undertaken with public funds at traditional academic institutions. In industry, projects generally involve many layers of oversight, and teams often specialize in and are responsible for particular methods or stages of the work. Yet, even large-scale science projects undertaken in collaboration with industry or through industry consortia may experience organizational difficulties if they require groups to mesh dissimilar organizational schemes and cultures.

Personnel Issues

The challenges involved in organizing and managing a large-scale science project include questions of staffing and the training of junior scientists working on the project. As mentioned above, much of the work in academic research laboratories is done by graduate students and postdoctoral fellows who are striving to build a scientific reputation and career. This is viewed as a mutually beneficial arrangement because students and fellows provide an inexpensive but highly effective labor pool in exchange for training and future career opportunities based on professional recognition for the publications they produce. However, this academic career track may not mesh well with the goals, products, and timeframe of many large-scale projects. Students who are assigned to work on a small piece of a large project may spend many years making a valuable contribution, but emerge without a significant publication record on which to base their career advancement. They may also fail to derive the crucial breadth of training or experience students obtain by working on and developing a smaller, independent project. As a result, it may be most appropriate to rely more on technical staff than on students when undertaking a long-term, product-oriented large-scale project.

Information Sharing and Intellectual Property Concerns

The success of big-science projects in fields such as high-energy physics has been attributed in part to the fact that the products of the research have no commercial value, and thus the scientists involved in a project are quite willing to share results and information (Kevles and Hood, 1992). In contrast, many large-scale projects in biomedical research have substantial commercial value, making it less likely that data and reagents will be freely shared. The potential profits to be gained in developing new drugs or other medically applicable technologies are enormous, and many products of large-scale projects can be used as tools in the development of such drugs and technologies. However, when many different research tools are needed to develop a clinically applicable product, aggressive enforcement of patents and pursuit of licensing revenues associated with those tools could potentially hamper the progress of research. As a result, there have been many debates about access to biological data and the merit and appropriate use of patenting and licensing of research tools in biomedicine (NIH, 1998; Heller and Eisenberg, 1998). The challenge is to strike a balance between patent protection and public access so that institutions are willing to take the risks and make the commitments necessary to develop new products with medical and commercial value without significantly impeding the progress of research in the field as a whole.

Projects funded by federal agencies may be more apt than those funded by private industry to rapidly place results into publicly accessible databases and to forego the potential revenues of patenting and licensing the products of the research. Again, however, there are no absolute distinctions between publicly and privately funded research with regard to these issues (Eisenberg, 2000). For example, some projects funded largely by industry consortia (such as the Single Nucleotide Polymorphisms [SNP] Consortium[1]) have policies regarding the creation of unencumbered public-domain database resources similar to those of the publicly funded HGP. On the other hand, legislation[2] passed in 1980 has encouraged academic scientists and others with federal funding to patent their findings in order to facilitate commercial development of the research.

SUMMARY

The ultimate goal of biomedical research, both large- and small-scale, is to advance knowledge and provide useful innovations to society. Determining the best and most efficient method for accomplishing that goal, however, is a continuing and evolving challenge. A review and assessment of large-scale science in biomedical research is warranted at this time because it is a relatively new concept in bioscience in general, and there is great interest in applying this scientific approach to address questions in the study of cancer. For the first time, scientists now have the ability to develop a large infrastructure upon which to base future research. The availability of genome sequences (human as well as model organisms, such as bacteria, yeast, worm, fruit fly, and mouse) allows for gene identification, examination of the regulation of gene expression, cross-species comparisons, and the study of polymorphisms in populations. Messenger RNA profiles can be generated to study the normal function and pathology of different tissues. Technology is available to study the structure and function of proteins, and their dependence on chemical modification and location within cells. Further improvements in experimental technologies and the informatics tools needed to process the information they generate will likely continue to enhance the speed and scale with which these resources can be generated and put to use.

When is a large-scale approach suitable for biomedical research, and what can we do to facilitate such efforts when they are deemed appropriate? The goals of this report are to examine the potential contributions of large-scale science to biomedical research, to identify impediments to applying the large-scale approach effectively, and to recommend ways of improving the process for future endeavors should they be undertaken.

---

[1] The SNP Consortium is composed of the Wellcome Trust and 11 pharmaceutical and technological companies: APBiotech, AstraZeneca PLC, Aventis, Bayer AG, Bristol-Meyers Squibb Company, F. Hoffmann-LaRoche, Glaxo Wellcome PLC, IBM, Motorola, Novartis, Pfizer Inc., Searle, and SmithKline Beecham PLC. See <http://snp.cshl.org/>.

[2] The Bayh-Dole Act and the Stevenson-Wydler Technology Innovation Act encouraged organizations to retain certain patent rights in government-sponsored research, and permitted the funded entity to transfer the technology to third parties. For more detail, see Chapter 7.

3

Models of Large-Scale Science

To further elaborate on the concept of large-scale biomedical science as defined in this report, this chapter provides an overview of several examples of past and current large-scale projects or strategies in biology and other fields. It begins with a summary of the Human Genome Project (HGP), the largest and most visible large-scale science project in biology to date. Many examples are drawn from NCI, in part because NCI has a longer history and more extensive ex-perience with directed, large-scale projects compared to other branches of NIH, and also because a major focus of this report is on cancer research. Several initiatives recently launched by other branches of NIH are described in detail, followed by examples of National Science Foundation (NSF) programs, industry consortia, public–private collaborations, and initiatives sponsored by private foundations. The chapter concludes with an example of a nonbiology model of large-scale science for contrast—that of the Defense Advanced Research Projects Agency (DARPA). The DARPA model is commonly cited as a potential strategy for undertaking large-scale, high-risk, and goal-oriented research, but this model has rarely been replicated in biology. A review of federally funded large-scale research projects in nonbiology fields such as high-energy physics is provided in the Appendix.

The common theme among the examples described in this chapter is that they are all formal programs launched by funding agencies, foundations, or industry. There is certainly no shortage of other ideas for potential large-scale biomedical research projects among scientists. Without an initiative by a funder, however, individual scientists may find it very difficult to obtain the funding necessary to launch an expensive, long-term, large-scale project because of the nature of traditional funding mechanisms (see Chapter 4).

Another common thread among these projects is their dependence on new or developing technologies. Technical innovations drive scientific discovery and determine what can be accomplished in the field. The pace and variety of new innovations have increased greatly in recent years, in turn increasing the feasibility of and opportunities for large-scale projects in biology (see Box 3-1). For example, the advent of DNA arrays and the development of software for analyzing the data they generate have made it feasible to study the entire transcriptional profiles of cells in health and disease or under various conditions. However, such projects are not only much larger in scale, but also much more expensive to undertake.

BOX 3-1   Examples of Important Technical Innovations in Biomedical Research

Many of the recent examples listed below are still in the early stages of development and have not yet demonstrated their full potential. These innovations are a driving force behind scientific advances and discoveries. The pace of innovation has accelerated in recent years, and many of the newer innovations could facilitate large-scale biology research initiatives.

1953   DNA structure elucidated
1960s   Genetic code deciphered
1970s   Restriction enzymes purified
        First cloned gene
        DNA sequencing methods developed
        Monoclonal antibodies produced
Today   Genome sequencing
        Computational algorithms
        SNP maps and human genetics
        Transcriptional profiles (assess all known genes in any normal or patho-
            logical tissue)
        Mass spectroscopy analysis of proteins
        Structural genomics (identification of all protein folds and domains, pre-
            diction of unknown protein structures)
        Combinatorial chemistry libraries
        Elucidation of signal transduction pathways involved in the development
            of cancer
        Structural biology–based drug design
        Chips for measuring protein activity
        High-volume pathological assessment (tissue arrays for normal and can-
            cer samples)

THE HUMAN GENOME PROJECT

Ever since the discoveries of genetic inheritance and the chemical structure of DNA, there has been interest in "unlocking the secrets of life" by deciphering the information encoded in the genome. Initially, scientists concentrated on small pieces of the puzzle because they lacked the ability to investigate genetic material efficiently on a large scale. As technological advances were made, however,[1] some molecular biologists began to discuss the feasibility and potential value of mapping and sequencing the entire human genome (see Figure 3-1). The first editorial published in a major scientific journal advocating a large-scale approach to sequence the human genome brought the concept to the scientific mainstream, with an emphasis on cancer research (Dulbecco, 1986). Nobel laureate Renato Dulbecco suggested that a project to map the human genome was the best way to make progress in the "war on cancer," which had been launched by the Nixon Administration in 1971. Dulbecco compared the significance of such a project to that of the U.S. space program, arguing that a genomic approach would facilitate a greater understanding of the genetic changes that lead to cancer, which would be essential in eradicating the disease. But he also noted that research on other diseases would certainly benefit as well.

At about the same time, a number of influential scientists were publicly discussing and advocating the possibility of sequencing the entire human genome (reviewed by Sulston and Ferry, 2002; Davies, 2001; Cook-Deegan, 1994, Kevles and Hood, 1992). In May 1985, Robert Sinsheimer, chancellor of the University of California Santa Cruz and a well-known molecular biologist, brought together a group of leading American and European molecular biologists to discuss the technical prospects for a human genome project. At this symposium on DNA sequencing, one of the strongest advocates for a large-scale HGP was Walter Gilbert, a Nobel laureate from Harvard, who had developed one of the first methods for sequencing DNA.

The following year, in early March 1986, Charles DeLisi, director of the Office of Health and Environmental Research at the U.S. Department of Energy (DOE), held a workshop to discuss the idea of undertaking an HGP under DOE. Although DOE may not have appeared to be the logical choice of a federal agency to oversee such a project, it had a long-standing research program on the effects of radiation on mutation rates, and the Life Sciences Division at Los Alamos National Laboratory had already established Genbank, a major database for DNA sequences, in 1983. DOE

---

[1] These technical advances included recombinant DNA methods, DNA sequencing methods, techniques for genetic mapping, and computer analysis.

May 1985	-- Robert Sinsheimer, UCSC chancellor hosts a meeting to discuss the technical prospects of the HGP.
March 1986	-- Editorial by Renato Dulbecco suggests that the HGP is the best way to make progress in the War on Cancer.
March 1986	-- Charles DeLisi holds a workshop to discuss the possibility of a DOE-sponsored HGP.
May 1986	-- A molecular biology meeting at Cold Spring Harbor includes a special session to discuss the possibility of the HGP.
February 1988	-- A report from the U.S. National Research Council endorses the HGP.
April 1988	-- The Congressional Office of Technology Assessment endorses the HGP.
September 1988	-- NIH establishes the Office of Human Genome Research, with James Watson as its head.
October 1989	-- The new NIH office becomes the National Center for Human Genome Research (NCHGR).
April 1990	-- NIH and DOE publish a 5-year mapping and sequencing plan, with a projected budget of $200 million/year.
1991	-- NIH funds ~175 genome projects, with an average grant size of ~$300,000/year.
July 1991	-- Craig Venter, then at NIH, reveals that NIH has applied for patents on expressed sequence tags (ESTs) identified by his laboratory.
April 1992	-- Watson resigns as head of NCHGR. Francis Collins appointed as his replacement in 1993.
June 1992	-- Venter leaves NIH to set up The Institute for Genomic Research (TIGR), a non-profit devoted to identifying human genes using EST methods.
October 1993	-- NIH and DOE publish a revised 5-year plan, with full completion expected in 2005.
October 1993	-- The Wellcome Trust and the U.K. Medical Research Council open the Sanger Center to sequence the human genome and model organisms.
September 1994	-- French and American researchers publish a complete genetic linkage map of the human genome, one year ahead of schedule.
December 1995	-- Another group of American and French scientists publishes a physical map of the human genome containing 15,000 marker sequences.
February 1996	-- International HGP partners agree to release sequence data into public databases within 24 hours.
January 1997	-- NCHGR renamed as National Human Genome Research Institute (NHGRI).
October 1997	-- Only 3 percent of the human genome is sequenced in finished form by the projected midway point of the 15-year HGP.
1998	-- ABI PRISM 3700 automated sequencing machines enter the laboratory market.
May 1998	-- Craig Venter announces formation of a company, later named Celera, to sequence the human genome in 3 years, using the whole genome shotgun approach.
May 1998	-- The Wellcome Trust announces that it will double its support for the HGP.
May 1998	-- Collins redirects the bulk of available NHGRI funds to three sequencing centers.
October 1998	-- NIH and DOE publish new goals for 1998-2003, expecting a working draft of the genome by 2003, and a full sequence by 2005.
March 1999	-- NIH moves the expected date for release of a working draft ahead to spring of 2000.
March 2000	-- Celera and academic collaborators release a draft sequence of the fruit fly genome, obtained using the whole-genome shotgun method.
March 2000	-- Possibility for collaboration between Celera and the public HGP wanes. Disagreement over data access is a major obstacle.
June 2000	-- HGP and Celera jointly announce a working draft of the human genome sequence.

FIGURE 3-1   A timeline of the human genome project.
SOURCE: Adapted from Macilwain (2000:983–4).

was also accustomed to big-science projects involving sophisticated technologies. It tended to oversee big, bureaucratic, goal-oriented projects, in contrast to the smaller, hypothesis-driven research that was the standard at NIH. DeLisi, formerly chief of mathematical biology at NIH, had been exploring the feasibility of such a project, and in 1986 he proposed a plan for a 5-year DOE HGP that would comprise physical mapping, development of automated high-speed sequencing, and research into computer analysis of sequence data.

Soon after, in May 1986, a meeting on molecular biology hosted by James Watson at Cold Spring Harbor included a special session dedicated to discussing the possibility of an HGP. During this session, Walter Gilbert estimated the cost of sequencing the human genome at $3 billion (approximately $1 per base). Many scientists opposed the endeavor on the basis of cost, as they assumed it would take funding away from other projects. The project was also viewed by many as a forced transition away from hypothesis-driven science to a directed, hierarchical mode of big science. Many argued that sequencing efforts should focus on the genes rather than the entire genome, which included large areas of repetitive DNA of unknown function. Searching for and characterizing genes hypothesized to be associated with human diseases was thought by opponents of the project to be the more scientifically valid approach than "blindly sequencing" the genome. However, advocates for the project argued that a large-scale HGP would be a less risky undertaking than big-science programs in space or physics. A failed space mission or particle accelerator would be extremely expensive and would be unlikely to yield partial benefits. In contrast, accomplishing even some of the goals of the HGP (e.g., an incomplete map or a partial sequence) would likely be very beneficial. Others suggested, however, that such a project would not advance medical science, because knowing the sequence of a gene does not necessarily foster progress in developing new treatments. For example, the single base-change mutation responsible for sickle cell anemia has been known for more than 20 years, but no therapies based on this knowledge have yet been developed. Many biologists also viewed DOE's efforts as a means of expanding its influence and involvement in biological research, as there were questions at the time about the future of the National Laboratories, given the volatility of national defense and energy policy since the 1970s (Cook-Deegan, 1994). They argued that a federally funded large-scale HGP, if undertaken at all, should be carried out through NIH.

One incentive for undertaking a federally funded HGP was to maintain a U.S. lead in biotechnology. In the late 1980s, genome efforts were gaining momentum in several other countries as well (reviewed by

Davies, 2001; Cook-Deegan, 1994; Kevles and Hood, 1992, Sulston and Ferry, 2002). In 1988, the European Community proposed the launch of a European Human Genome Project. A modified proposal was adopted in 1989, authorizing a 3-year commitment of 15 million euros, 7 percent of which would be devoted to ethical issues. Meanwhile, human genome programs at the national level were also prospering in Europe. For example, in 1989 the British government committed itself to a formal human genome program, funded at 11 million pounds per year for the first 3 years. In France, the Centre d'Etude du Polymorphisme Humain (CEPH), a key player in developing the genetic linkage map of the human genome, was founded by Nobelist Jean Dausset with funds from a scientific award and gifts from a private French donor. Through additional support from the Howard Hughes Medical Institute (HHMI), CEPH made clones of its DNA available to dozens of researchers in Europe, North America, and Africa. Japan, which had thus far been involved only marginally in biotechnology research, was also pushing hard to develop new automated sequencing technologies, with the objective of a major sequencing initiative. In 1988, the international Human Genome Organization (HUGO) was formed, primarily with funding from HHMI and the Imperial Cancer Research Fund in Great Britain (Kevles and Hood, 1992). Its goal was to help coordinate human genome research internationally; to foster exchanges of data, materials, and technologies; and to encourage genomic studies of organisms other than human beings, such as mice.

Because of the controversies surrounding the proposed U.S. HGP, the National Research Council (NRC) was commissioned to undertake a study to determine a strategy for the project. The NRC study, chaired by Bruce Alberts, generated a report (NRC, 1988) advocating an international program led by the United States and containing the following recommendations:

- Postponing large-scale sequencing until the necessary technology could be improved, thereby reducing the cost per base (estimated to be about a 5-year delay)
- Making technology development for sequencing a high priority
- Focusing first on mapping the human genome
- Characterizing the genomes of model organisms (e.g., mouse, fruit fly, yeast, bacteria)
- Providing $200 million in funding per year for up to 15 years

The report did not make a recommendation as to whether the NIH or DOE should oversee the project. In 1988, however, NIH and DOE reached an agreement on their working relationship for the next 5 years: NIH would primarily map the chromosomes, while DOE would develop technologies and informatics, with collaboration occurring between the two agencies in overlapping areas.

In 1988, DeLisi submitted a budget from DOE of $12 million. In the same year, NIH Director James Wyngaarden offered James Watson, Nobel laureate and codiscoverer of the helical structure of DNA, the position of associate director of human genome research. Watson built political support for the project, and made a commitment to devote about 5 percent of its budget to the study of the project's ethical, legal, and social implications.[2] In October 1989, the unit became the National Center for Human Genome Research, with a budget of $60 million for fiscal year 1990 (Davies, 2001).

The HGP actually entailed three related endeavors: genetic mapping, physical mapping, and sequencing. Genetic mapping is accomplished by determining the order and approximate location of genetic markers, such as genes and polymorphisms, on each chromosome. Physical mapping involves breaking each chromosome into small, ordered, overlapping fragments and placing these fragments into vectors that can easily be stored and replicated. For the sequencing phase, fragments of each chromosome are processed to determine the base pair code.[3]

The U.S. HGP was inaugurated as a formal federal program in 1991, receiving about $135 million. Seven NIH centers were involved: five focused on human gene mapping, one focused on mouse gene mapping, and one focused on yeast chromosome sequencing. These centers were supported on a competitive, peer-reviewed basis. In 1991, the largest center budget was $4 million, divided among several research groups. The genome installations at DOE's National Laboratories were focused on developing technologies for mapping, sequencing, and informatics. Four additional projects, funded jointly by NIH and DOE, were engaged in large-scale sequencing efforts and innovations. In addition, dozens of smaller, investigator-initiated gene mapping and sequencing projects aimed at single disease-associated genes were funded by NIH in laboratories across the country. For example, in 1991 NIH funded about 175 different genome projects, with an average grant size of $312,000 a year (about 1.5 times the average grant size for basic research, and about equal to the average AIDS research grant). Thus, the HGP initially was characterized more by loose coordination, local freedom, and programmatic and insti-

---

[2] This commitment of NIH funds to ethical debate was unprecedented, as was making bioethics an integral part of an NIH biological research program.

[3] The original plan called for carefully orchestrated sequencing of the fragments derived from physical mapping; more recently, however, a "shotgun" method has been used to sequence random fragments from a chromosome, followed by application of computer algorithms to determine the order of the sequence fragments.

tutional pluralism than by strong central management or external hierarchy (Kevles and Hood, 1992).

Criticism of the program continued, however, especially with regard to funding priorities at NIH. During the late 1980s, the proportion of grants funded by NIH fell from 40 percent to less than 25 percent (Davis, 1990). For example, the National Institute for General Medical Sciences (NIGMS) awarded more than 900 new and competing renewal grants for projects unrelated to the genome in 1988; in 1990, it awarded only 550, a 43 percent decrease. Across NIH, the total number of grants had fallen from 6000 to 4,600 a year (fewer than the number funded in 1981). This drop caused great consternation among biomedical scientists, and many assumed that it was due directly to the transfer of funds to the HGP, though close examination of concurrent changes in NIH funding patterns suggests that this was not the case. In the mid-1980s, the average grant period was extended from 3.3 to 4.3 years to provide greater stability for funded projects and reduce the frequency of grant applications; the average amount of funding per grant also increased significantly. But this in turn reduced the funds available for new awards or renewals. During the same period, the production of Ph.D. scientists in the field of biomedicine greatly increased, so more people were competing for grant money. Supporters of the HGP argued that the project was bringing appropriations to biomedical research that simply would not otherwise have been received. In any case, NIH expenditures on the project in 1991 accounted for only 1 percent of the agency's total budget of $8 billion (Kevles and Hood, 1992).

In addition, the project's deliberate emphasis on technological and methodological innovation was contrary to the tradition and preference of many in the biomedical research community. However, much progress in biomedical science has been fostered and accelerated by sophisticated tools and technologies, often those developed through work in other fields, such as the physical sciences (Varmus, 1999). Furthermore, unlike technologies in the field of high-energy physics, those in biology tend to become smaller, cheaper, and more widely obtainable and dispersed as they improve. Thus technology development in biology is more likely to benefit a large number of scientists in the long run, rather than making the field more exclusive.

The HGP faced a new challenge in 1992 when James Watson resigned. Earlier that year, a controversy had arisen regarding patent applications on gene fragments. J. Craig Venter, who was working at NIH at the time, had used a high-throughput technique for sequencing fragments of genes from cDNA libraries (known as expressed sequence tags, or ESTs). NIH applied for patents on hundreds of ESTs on Venter's behalf. The patents were eventually rejected by the Patent Office on the grounds that they did not meet the criteria of nonobviousness, novelty, and utility. Initial rejection of an application is not unusual, and NIH had the option to appeal the decision, but in 1994 a decision was made to abandon the effort. These patent applications were widely criticized by the scientific community at large, and the issues surrounding DNA patents continue to be controversial.

Francis Collins was appointed in 1993 to be Watson's successor. Collins had been among the first to identify a human disease gene (for cystic fibrosis) through positional cloning, a technique that relies on genetic and physical mapping. By the time of his new appointment, he had also been involved in the discovery of several additional disease genes[4] using similar methods.

The HGP soon faced new criticism. By 1997, the midpoint of the 15-year project, only 3 percent of the human genome had been sequenced in finished form, and there were many technical difficulties with the physical maps of the chromosomes (Rowen et al., 1997; Anderson, 1993). Although the first 6 years of the project had deliberately focused on smaller genomes and on the development of techniques that would allow for a more efficient and cost-effective approach to large-scale sequencing of the human genome, sequencing technologies had not yet been sufficiently improved to either dramatically speed the sequencing process or reduce the cost (Pennisi, 1998). As a result, there was concern about whether the project could be completed within the projected timeframe or budget.

In 1998, the technology of DNA sequencing took a major step forward when the Applied Biosystems Incorporated (ABI) PRISM 3700 entered the laboratory market (Davies, 2001; Wade, 2001). While not the first automated sequencer, the ABI PRISM was still an evolutionary advance over existing commercial automation because it provided increased capacity and throughput. It incorporated two major modifications to the original Sanger sequencing method: it used fluorescent dyes instead of radioactivity to label the DNA fragments, so that a laser detector and computer could identify and record each letter in the sequence as the DNA fragments were eluted; and it separated DNA fragments in ultrathin capillary tubes filled with a polymer solution, rather than the traditional polyacrylamide slab gels. These improvements were the inspiration of Michael Hunkapiller, and the machines were produced by ABI, originally an independent company that had been purchased by the scientific instrument maker Perkin-Elmer (PE) and now a subsidiary of Applera. As a result of these technological advances, DNA samples could be separated much more quickly, and several samples could be processed each day using very small volumes of reagents. The new machines required only about 15 minutes of human intervention every 24 hours, compared with 8 hours

---

[4] The genes for neurofibromatosis 1 and Huntington's disease.

for the traditional machine. These changes cut sequencing time by 60 percent, reduced labor costs by 90 percent, and produced sequence about eight times faster (about 1 million bases a day) than traditional sequencing methods (Davies, 2001).

The new sequencing machines were used early on by Craig Venter, who had left NIH in 1992 to found The Institute for Genomic Research (TIGR), a nonprofit organization devoted initially to identifying expressed human genes using EST methods. The organization had since branched out into other areas of genomic research, such as sequencing the genomes of bacteria. It was also a major player in the federally funded HGP. TIGR was the first center to use and verify the effectiveness of the "shotgun" method for sequencing the relatively small, simple genomes of microbes. The advent of the new sequencing machines led Hunkapiller to consider the possibility of rapidly sequencing the entire human genome using a similar approach, and he brought the idea to Venter. In 1998, Venter left TIGR to found Celera, initially an independent subsidiary of PE Corporation and now a subsidiary of Applera—the same company that produced the ABI PRISM 3700 sequencing machines—with the goal of doing just that.

The feasibility of such a project was widely questioned in the scientific community. The PRISM sequencers were still largely untested, and the shotgun method had never been used on anything other than bacterial genomes. Many predicted that the final product would likely have many more gaps and errors than would result from the methodical approach of the public project because of the size, repetitiveness, and complexity of mammalian genomes as compared with microbial genomes. Venter and colleagues (1998) argued that these challenges could be overcome, and Celera launched a test project to sequence the genome of the fruit fly *Drosophila*, a complex eukaryote whose genome was about one-twentieth the size of the human genome. It took Celera 4 months to prepare a rough sequence draft of the *Drosophila* genome, suggesting that the human genome could be deciphered in this way as well (Loder, 2000; Pennisi, 2000a).

To accomplish the goal of producing a complete rough draft of the human genome sequence by 2001 (4 years ahead of the public project's timetable), Celera purchased about 300 PRISM 3700 sequencers and a supercomputer for sequence analysis. The company also recruited a large number of people who specialized in developing algorithms and software for sifting through and organizing the huge amounts of data to be generated. Most notable was Gene Myers, who had already been working on shotgun assembly algorithms at the University of Arizona. Venter estimated that the total cost to sequence the human genome would be about $200–500 million. By this time, $1.9 billion had already been invested in the publicly funded HGP, but questions were raised as to whether Celera's efforts would now make continuation of the public project redundant and unnecessary. On the other hand, supporters of the public project believed the new challenge from Celera was ample reason to accelerate the public effort. Some of the concern stemmed from the potential commercial exploitation of genomic data, although the company had announced that it would seek patents on only 100–300 genes. The Celera business plan entailed selling access to sequence analysis, such as information on gene identification, DNA variants, medical relevance, and comparisons with other species. Celera still planned to release raw sequence data free of charge, but only every 3 months, as opposed to every 24 hours as in the public project (Davies, 2001).

Shortly after the launch of Celera, the Wellcome Trust doubled support for the Sanger Center, Great Britain's main sequencing center in the public effort. Francis Collins also suggested producing a public rough draft of the sequence first, by 2001, to coincide with Celera's target date. The public consortium would then release a finished, "gold-standard" version by the original deadline in 2004, a goal that Celera had never established. To meet this new deadline, Collins redirected the bulk of available NIH funds to just three centers, announcing that these three centers would receive $80 million over 5 years. At about the same time, the Wellcome Trust announced that it would provide another $7 million to the Sanger Center. Thus the lion's share of the draft sequence would be produced by five major genome centers: Sanger, three centers funded by NIH (Whitehead Institute, Washington University, and Baylor College of Medicine), and DOE's Joint Genome Institute. To meet the new goal, hundreds of PRISM sequencers (or similar machines) were purchased by the publicly funded centers (Davies, 2001).

The competition and animosity between the public and private efforts to sequence the genome escalated (reviewed by Davies, 2001; Wade, 2001), but as the self-imposed deadline to finish the draft sequence approached, a compromise was brokered between the leaders of the two projects. On June 26, 2000, Craig Venter and Francis Collins came together for a White House press conference to formally announce completion of the draft sequence. The first publications on the draft sequences were published about 7 months later in the journals *Nature* and *Science* (Lander et al., 2001; Venter et al., 2001). *Science* has been criticized for its decision to publish Celera's analysis because the company was allowed to post its data in its own database with some restrictions on its use, rather than depositing the sequence into a public database such as Genbank, as is usually required for publication. Leaders of the public project have also noted that Celera's analysis was dependent upon access to the public databases, suggesting that the company's shotgun method alone could not have produced an assembled sequence of high quality (Waterston et al., 2002a).

The public consortium has continued its efforts to analyze the sequence and to fill in gaps and correct errors; completion of the finished version was announced in April 2003 (Pennisi, 2003). However, the rough draft sequence is now freely available to any biomedical scientist in the world. Recently, a draft of the mouse genome was also published (Waterston et al., 2002b). These sequences provide a rich resource for biomedical research. The process of identifying disease-related genes, once an expensive and arduous undertaking, has become a rapid, highly automated process limited primarily by access to the relevant human populations. Of course, the lag time between finding a gene and developing a clinically relevant therapy for a disease is still likely to be quite long. Nonetheless, the completion of the HGP has accelerated the pace of biomedical discovery. The sequence is likely to have an equally dramatic effect on other areas of basic biological research, such as evolutionary biology.

The HGP's goal of producing a powerful research tool has been met, in spite of the criticism and controversy surrounding the project. Knowledge of the human sequence, as well as those of model organisms, has already greatly facilitated basic research in such areas as microarray analysis and proteomics. There is also, as noted, great hope for developing clinical applications of the new knowledge to directly advance human health. Questions may still be raised, however, as to whether the project was carried out in the most effective and efficient manner, or even whether competition from the private sector was a positive force in finishing the project. With the completion of the HGP has come an increased interest in taking on additional publicly funded large-scale biology projects. Thus, these are important questions to address when considering a new large-scale undertaking in biomedical science.

PAST EXAMPLES OF LARGE-SCALE PROJECTS FUNDED BY NCI

Three large-scale programs developed by NCI in the 1950s and 1960s while perhaps not strictly meeting the working definition of large-scale science used for this report, may prove instructive in understanding some of the issues relevant to NCI's more recent large-scale initiatives. Although NCI's extramural grants program, like those of most branches of NIH, has supported mostly investigator-initiated projects funded on the basis of scientific peer review, a markedly different approach was used for much of the research carried out under these three programs—in Cancer Chemotherapy, Chemical Carcinogenesis, and Cancer Viruses. Each of these programs entailed large-scale, directed research and often employed the contract funding mechanism, with comparatively little input from and control by the scientific community; rather, NCI staff assumed responsibility for the programs and had authority over the assignment of research contracts to investigators (reviewed by Rettig, 1977). Over time, contract research grew to be a substantial portion of the NCI budget, about 80 percent of which was devoted to these three directed programs in 1971 (U.S. Department of Health, Education, and Welfare, 1973).

Cancer Chemotherapy Program

The cancer chemotherapy program was launched in 1955. During World War II, it was discovered that nitrogen mustard could induce temporary remissions in certain forms of leukemia and lymphoma, and this discovery led to the search for additional chemical agents for cancer treatment. The methodical search for chemotherapeutics took place in multiple stages. First, a large number of chemical compounds were procured and screened for antitumor effects. Promising compounds were then evaluated for toxicity, first in animals and then in humans. Finally, compounds were tested in human clinical trials for therapeutic effect. Between 1955 and the late 1970s, more than 500,000 chemicals were tested on laboratory animals in NCI's chemotherapy program. Several hundred of these chemicals had also been tested in clinical trials, and about 45 chemicals had been found to have some effect against 29 forms of cancer (DeVita and Goldin, 1984).

One of the great challenges for the program was establishing the protocols and appropriate animal models for screening the antitumor effects of compounds. Early on, the contract research system appeared to be a logical approach for large-scale screening of chemicals, especially given the substantial need for animal production facilities. Administrative integration of the program components was less complicated using a centrally managed contract system as opposed to a more traditional program of extramural grants. A large portion of the contract work was actually performed by private industrial firms.

For many years, this program was the subject of great controversy within the scientific community, dividing scientists committed to fundamental research and those with a focus on targeted or directed research. The program was widely criticized for its dependence on contract research and its lack of communication with the scientific community. Indeed, a 1965 White House report, commissioned to determine whether Americans were getting their money's worth from NIH-sponsored medical research, singled out the cancer chemotherapy program for harsh criticism. The report noted that many medical scientists had questioned whether the cost of the program could be justified by its output. The review group for the program concluded that a substantial fraction of the contract work done within the program was of relatively low scientific quality and showed evidence of inadequate central supervision (U.S. President's NIH Study Committee, 1965).

Another independent committee was appointed by the secretary of Health, Education and Welfare in 1966 to review the funding of NIH research, including the cancer chemotherapy program. Chaired by Jack Ruina, who had extensive experience with grant and contract support of research and development in the Department of Defense, the committee concluded that the grant mechanism was inappropriate for directed research and development programs, and that contracts should be used instead. Nonetheless, the scientific community continued to express dissatisfaction with NCI's directed research efforts. The committee's report stated that plans for directed research, including objectives, justification, expected funding levels, management plans, and types of contractors, should be submitted to an appropriate advisory council for review and approval prior to a program's initiation, termination, or substantial change in scale or direction. The committee recommended, however, that once a program had been initiated, a program manager take full responsibility for its execution and oversight. The committee further urged NIH to take significant steps to make career opportunities and status for program managers more attractive. Moreover, it recommended that the practice of using intramural scientists to oversee directed research be replaced with a strong, independent management structure (U.S. Department of Health, Education and Welfare, 1966). In spite of this last recommendation, however, NCI staff who managed the directed research programs also continued to have responsibility for related aspects of the intramural program because of the difficulty in recruiting outside scientific talent to assume these management roles. This situation led to conflicts regarding the promotion and tenure of intramural research staff (Rettig, 1977). The staff's administrative responsibilities for the directed research programs reduced the amount of time they could spend on the conduct of their own research; thus they often published fewer papers than scientists from other branches of NIH. Because the traditional criteria for promotion and tenure stressed productivity in the form of published scientific articles, NCI staff members were often at a disadvantage in tenure and promotion decisions, which were reviewed collectively by the scientific directors of all the NIH institutes.

In 1975 the cancer chemotherapy program was combined with the surgery and radiation branches of NCI to form the Clinical Oncology Program (DeVita and Goldin, 1984). The development of therapeutic agents continues to be a focus of NCI's Developmental Therapeutics Program (DTP). Among the chemical compounds that have been slated for clinical development since at least 1981, 13 have been approved by the U.S. Food and Drug Administration (FDA).[5] According to a 1995 report (known as the Bishop-Calebresi report) that reviewed NCI's intramural program and was undertaken at the request of then-director Richard Klausner, this program has become an international resource, available to academic and commercial investigators alike (National Cancer Advisory Board, 1995). However, the report criticized the program for being intellectually isolated and underutilized by both the intramural and extramural communities of NCI, in part because of a failure to reach out to the larger community of scientists. The report further criticized the program for a lack of flexibility in its tactics and strategies, and identified problems with accountability and review. NCI has since initiated a new program called Rapid Access to Intervention (RAID). The goal of RAID[6] is to speed up the preclinical testing for promising drugs by targeting academic laboratories that have novel candidate compounds, but lack the specific resources or expertise needed to develop them further.

Chemical Carcinogenesis Program

NCI's second large-scale, directed program was launched in 1962. The goal of the chemical carcinogenesis program was to evaluate suspected chemical compounds for their cancer-causing properties, using one of two approaches: the first was to analyze occupation settings in which humans were known to be exposed to measurable amounts of specific chemicals; the second was to undertake epidemiological studies to ascertain major differences in the forms and incidence of cancer among various locations and cultures. Of the three NCI programs discussed here, chemical carcinogenesis received the least amount of funding and attention, and was not remarkably productive. The criteria for determining whether a given chemical is carcinogenic were (and still are) very difficult to establish, and a major obstacle to overcome was again the development of biological tests or models that could predict carcinogenic effects in humans. The undertaking was also seen as potentially leading to conflict with and regulation of the chemical industry, which was not the usual purview of NCI (Rettig, 1977).

The research efforts under the program were run by project officers who were trained as research scientists. The project officers set up contracts with various extramural investigators to collaborate within the scope of their own research expertise, and they coauthored extramural

---

[5] See <http://dtp.nci.nih.gov/docs/idrugs/drugstatus.html> [accessed 1/02/03].
[6] See <http://dtp.nci.nih.gov/docs/raid/raid_pp.html>.

research publications. Contracts were reviewed by project officers, along with an advisory group, about once a month. The reviewers considered future needs in addition to examining the status of current research contracts.

In the late 1970s and early 1980s, extensive changes took place within the chemical carcinogenesis program. The first was that program officers were no longer permitted to be associated with extramural research projects. The review process was completely removed from within the individual intramural programs, and outside review was initiated. The officers still provided oversight for contracts, but could not provide any scientific input, and they were no longer included on extramural publications. The second major change was the separation of testing and basic research. The carcinogen-testing portion of the program was moved to the National Institute of Environmental Health Sciences (NIEHS) and was called the National Toxicology Program (NTP). The NTP is affiliated with FDA, and is funded jointly by FDA, the Centers for Disease Control and Prevention (CDC), and NIEHS (its current annual budget is $160 million). The NTP produces the Report on Carcinogens, a list of all substances that either are known to be human carcinogens or may reasonably be anticipated to be human carcinogens, and to which a significant number of people in the United States are exposed. However, the report does not present quantitative assessments of carcinogenic risk. Basic research in carcinogenesis is now funded through a branch within the Division of Cancer Biology. This basic research is supported by grants, and there are currently no large-scale projects.

Cancer Virus Program

NCI's third major contract program, the special virus cancer program, was established in 1964. Scientists knew that certain types of cancer in chickens and rodents could be induced by viruses, and this knowledge led to the hypothesis that viruses could also be cancer-causing agents in humans. The goal of the program was to identify such causative viruses and to develop preventive vaccines against them. Eventually, the contract mechanism for this program was replaced by the more traditional investigator-initiated grants, in large part because of scathing criticism in a report on how the contract research program was being run (Culliton, 1974; National Cancer Advisory Board, 1974). In particular, the report criticized the contract proposal process because it was dominated by program officials, included potential and actual contractors in the review of proposals, lacked scientific rigor, and was inaccessible to the larger virology community. In addition, the contract research program represented an extension of the intramural research work of some program scientists.

As a result of the report, the contract review process was modified to make it more open and rigorous (Rettig, 1977). The formal program ultimately faded away, but research on viruses was continued through other programs at NCI and NIH.

The cancer virus program could be considered a significant failure of directed research since it did not lead directly to the identification of any viruses that cause human cancer; however, it had many indirect, beneficial effects on the scientific community. Many viruses (mostly RNA viruses) were found to cause cancer in a variety of animals, but investigators had begun to doubt whether any human cancers could be linked to viruses. The first human leukemia virus (HTLV1) was then identified and characterized by two independent laboratories in the early 1980s (Yoshida et al., 1982; Gallo et al., 1982). Later, it was discovered that the Epstein-Barr virus (a DNA virus) could also cause human cancer. It is now known that two of the most common cancers in the worldwide population—cervical and liver cancer—are caused by virus infections (reviewed by Gallo, 1999). Furthermore, the recognition of viral oncogenes has led to the identification of cellular oncogenes and tumor suppressor genes, which play an important role in most non–virus-associated human cancers.

These discoveries did not result directly from the targeted research of the cancer virus program, but certainly were aided indirectly by the groundwork and scientific infrastructure developed by that program. An unintended but beneficial return on the investment in cancer virology was the development of technologies for the field of molecular biology—the purification and production of reverse transcriptase being a prime example. Research on human immunodeficiency virus (HIV) also benefited greatly from the work on retroviruses that was undertaken through the cancer virus program. Ironically, however, if technology development had been the stated goal of the program, it most likely would have received less funding. At the time the program was initiated, Congress and NIH were not very receptive to funding programs aimed simply at developing biological technologies. In the current environment, technology development may be a more acceptable goal in and of itself.

RECENTLY DEVELOPED LARGE-SCALE PROJECTS AT NCI

The Cancer Genome Anatomy Project

The Cancer Genome Anatomy Project (CGAP) is an interdisciplinary program established and administered by NCI to generate the information and technological tools needed to decipher the molecular anatomy of cancer cells. It was launched after extensive input had been gathered from a committee of external scientists who were considered leaders in the field of cancer biology. The goal of the CGAP is to achieve a comprehensive molecular characterization of normal, precancerous, and malignant cells in order to determine the molecular changes that occur when a normal cell is transformed into a cancer cell, and then to apply that knowledge to the prevention, detection, and management of cancer.[7] Since its inception in 1996, the program has encompassed four primary initiatives:

- The Human Tumor Gene Index—identifies genes expressed during the development of human tumors.
- The Cancer Chromosome Aberration Project—characterizes the chromosomal alterations associated with malignant transformation.
- The Genetic Annotation Index—identifies and characterizes the polymorphisms associated with cancer.
- The Mouse Tumor Gene Index—identifies genes expressed during the development of mouse tumors.

The goals of CGAP clearly overlap extensively with some of the goals of the HGP (for example, identifying expressed genes and using experimental high-throughput technologies). In fact, the director of CGAP was first hired by NIH to oversee technology initiatives for the HGP.[8] The program was started when NCI was becoming more open to administrative experimentation and to an approach to project management focused on solving problems. The program director reports directly to the NCI director, and is expected to move the field ahead as quickly as possible. This is a somewhat fragile arrangement as it depends on an NCI director who supports technology development, as well as an institutional culture that welcomes an aggressive program management style similar to the DARPA model (see page 74), with an openness to a directive, problem-solving funding mode that does not always rely on external peer review for project selection. The project includes both intramural and contract funding.

All data and materials from CGAP are shared openly and quickly with the research community without restrictions. The CGAP website includes databases containing genomic data for human and mouse, including ESTs, gene expression patterns, single nucleotide polymorphisms (SNPs), cluster assemblies, and cytogenetic information. Informatics tools to query and analyze the data are also developed by the program and made available online. In addition, NCI provides information on new experimental methods and makes biological reagents developed through the program available to researchers at cost.

---

[7] See <http://cgap.nci.nih.gov/>.
[8] Robert Strausberg, director of NCI's CGAP, in presentations to the National Cancer Policy Board.

Investigators funded through the program are required to sign an agreement stating that they will not patent the sequences they acquire. For sequencing projects, NCI has obtained a declaration of "exceptional circumstances" under the Bayh-Dole Act, meaning that contractors do not retain title to inventions developed with the federal funds. NCI is thereby able to mandate immediate disclosure of data by its contractors.

In the future, the program may become involved in the development of functional genomics and proteomics databases. The ultimate goal in any case is to develop tools and infrastructures for the scientific community.

Early Detection Research Network

The Early Detection Research Network (EDRN)[9] is a relatively new, large-scale program of the Cancer Biomarkers Research Group in the Division of Cancer Prevention at NCI. EDRN is a national network whose purpose is to establish a scientific consortium of investigators with resources for basic, translational, and clinical research aimed at developing, evaluating, and validating biomarkers for earlier cancer detection and risk assessment. The network was established in response to concerns in the field that bringing validated biomarkers into the clinic would require a pooling of resources and expertise. It encourages collaboration and rapid dissemination of information among investigators.

In an attempt to bridge the gap between laboratory advances and the clinical adoption of biomarkers, EDRN has brought organizations with varied interests and corporate cultures together in a single scientific consortium.[10] Because many steps are necessary to ensure that a marker is accurate, reproducible, and practical for medical application, the consortium is organized into four working and two oversight components. The working components are as follows:

• Biomarker Developmental Laboratories that identify, characterize, and refine techniques for finding molecular, genetic, and biologic signs of cancer

• Clinical and Epidemiological Centers that focus on providing the network with blood, tissue, other biological samples, and medical information on families with histories of cancer

• Biomarker Validation Laboratories that standardize tests and prepare them for clinical trials, serving as crucial intermediaries between the Biomarker Developmental Laboratories and clinical practice

---

[9] See <http://edrn.nci.nih.gov>.

[10] See <http://www.nih.gov/news/pr/May 20000/nci-16.htm>.

• A Data Management and Coordination Center to develop standards for data reporting and to study new statistical methods for analyzing biomarkers

The oversight components consist of a steering committee and an advisory committee. The steering committee provides major scientific management oversight, and has responsibility for developing and implementing protocols, designs, and operations. This committee determines which markers identified by the Biomarker Developmental Laboratories should advance to the Biomarker Validation Laboratories. Its members are principal investigators from the funded laboratories and centers, NCI program staff, and other ad hoc members invited by the committee. The advisory committee reviews the progress of the network, recommends new research initiatives, and ensures that the network is responsive to promising opportunities in early-detection research and risk assessment. Its members are predominantly investigators who are not in the EDRN.

Funding through the program is based on peer review, using criteria established by the steering committee to meet the objectives and needs of the EDRN. Collaborations between funded network investigators and investigators from U.S. and foreign institutes and industries are also encouraged. This type of collaboration is referred to as associate membership.

In 1999, NCI awarded nearly $8 million to create 18 Biomarker Developmental Laboratories.[11] They are searching for potential biomarkers by analyzing thousands of samples of breast, prostate, ovarian, lung, bladder, and other cancers. Nine of these 18 grantees are collaborating with industry. In the spring of 2000, EDRN awarded an additional $18 million in first-year funding for nine Clinical and Epidemiological Centers, three Biomarker Validation Laboratories, and the Data Management and Coordinating Center.

Unconventional Innovations Program

NCI's Office of Technology and Industrial Relations (OTIR) was established with the mission of speeding the progress of cancer research by encouraging the development of new technologies and promoting scientific collaborations between NCI and the private sector. It serves as a point of access to NCI for private industry and technology developers, and plays a key role in the management of several programs for NCI, including the Unconventional Innovations Program (UIP).[12] The UIP was

---

[11] See <http://newscenter.cancer.gov/>.
[12] See <http://otir.nci.nih.gov/otir/index.html>.

created in 1998 with the intent of fostering risky technology development to improve progress in cancer research, a goal that was not a traditional aim at NIH.[13] Specifically, the program sought technology platforms integrating noninvasive sensing of molecular alterations in vivo with transmission of information to an external monitor, controlled intervention specific for the molecular profile, and monitoring of the intervention. The program was targeted to invest $48 million over a 5-year period. The first five contracts were issued through the program in 1999, totaling about $11 million over 3 years. In 2000, four contracts were issued, totaling about $9 million over 3 years.

Before soliciting the first round of applications for UIP funding, NCI requested input on new opportunities for the detection and treatment of cancer at the earliest stages by calling for "white papers" describing those opportunities.[14] The interest and involvement of investigators from disciplines that have not traditionally received support from NCI were specifically recruited. Ideas and information submitted by investigators contributed to the development of the first Broad Agency Announcement (BAA) solicitation for the UIP in 1999.

A BAA stipulates technical goals but does not specify how to achieve them, so applicants are encouraged to propose different technological approaches. This mechanism is commonly used by DARPA (see page 74) and the Office of Naval Research, but it is an unusual approach within NIH. However, the selection process for UIP contracts, similar to most NIH funding mechanisms, is based on peer review. All proposals are evaluated by a peer review group known as the Technology Evaluation Panel, which considers four criteria: potential contribution and relevance to the UIP, technical approach, the applicant's capabilities, and plans and capability to accomplish technology maturation.

The management style of the UIP also resembles that of DARPA, involving continued interaction between NCI staff and awardees. Yearly meetings of principal investigators funded through the UIP are held to provide a forum for discussing progress, forging collaborations among investigators, showcasing complementary programs and resources, and soliciting feedback from investigators. (At NCI, convening of a planning group is common, but regular meetings of awardees are not commonly held.) One goal of these meetings is to bring together a critical mass of investigators in a particular area who might otherwise not communicate with each other.

The UIP clearly differs from the core scientific programs at NIH in

---

[13] Carol Dahl, former director of the NCI's Unconventional Innovations Program, in a presentation to the National Cancer Policy Board, July 16, 2002.

[14] See <http://amb.nci.nih.gov/> [accessed 1/10/00].

being focused on high-risk technology development, as opposed to hypothesis-driven research. An explicit mandate of the UIP is to develop enabling technologies and build infrastructure to advance an entire field, as well as to create new fields. The program objectives expressly call for the development of technologies that target quantum improvements in existing technologies or entirely new approaches, rather than incremental improvements to the state of the art.[15] The original request for white papers defined the ultimate goal of the program as follows:

> Building on the work of CGAP in molecular profiling of tumors, the NCI wishes to create technology platforms that will revolutionize cancer detection, diagnosis and treatment. The NCI is interested in identifying technology systems or components that will enable sensing of molecular alterations in the body in a way that is highly sensitive and specific, yet non-intrusive. The technology system should additionally serve as the platform for, or have a seamless integration with, capabilities for the intervention specific for the detected molecular profile. Building on this ambitious objective will require the development and integration of a series of capabilities including highly specific molecular recognition, signaling capability, controllable intervention capabilities, methods for monitoring intervention release and impact, and biotolerance. This will require the input and collaboration of investigators from a variety of disciplines, many of which have not traditionally engaged in cancer research.[16]

Although a number of papers have been published recently by the awardees of the program, it is still too early to measure the program's success. However, satisfaction with the progress of the program was sufficient for NCI to enter into a new collaboration with the National Aeronautics and Space Administration (NASA) for a project with goals that are complementary to those of the UIP. A joint NASA/NCI solicitation was released on January 3, 2001, to support fundamental technologies for the development of biomolecular sensors.

Mouse Models of Human Cancers Consortium

The Mouse Models of Human Cancers Consortium (MMHCC), assembled from multidisciplinary teams of scientists, was established in 1999 for the collaborative development, characterization, and validation of mouse models that parallel the ways in which human cancers develop,

---

[15] "This program seeks to stimulate development of radically new technologies in cancer care that can transform what is now impossible into the realm of the possible for detecting, diagnosing, and intervening in cancer at its earliest stages of development." See <http://otir.nci.nih.gov/tech/uip.html>.

[16] See <http://amb.nci.nih.gov/> [accessed 1/10/00].

progress, and respond to therapy or preventive agents. As in the case of CGAP, the MMHCC was launched with considerable input from the scientific community. One goal of the program is to define the standards by which to validate the models for their relevance to human cancer biology and for testing therapy, prevention, early detection, or diagnostic strategies. Ultimately, the Consortium is responsible for choosing which existing mouse cancer models warrant full characterization for their relevance to human cancer, and which new models should be derived and characterized when no model exists for a given malignancy.

The purpose of implementing the MMHCC was to accelerate the pace at which mouse models are made available to the research community for further investigation or application. The consortium enables interactions to foster the rapid exchange of ideas, information, and technology. NCI works with the consortium to organize workshops and symposia, to provide information about the models and related technology, and to plan for distribution of the validated mouse models to the cancer research community.

Funding for members of the MMHCC is available through both NIH intramural projects and the U01 funding mechanism (see Chapter 4 for an explanation of the various NIH funding mechanisms).[17] The program has thereby supported many small individual projects with grants similar in size to a typical R01 grant. However, the U01 mechanism is a cooperative agreement, in which substantial NCI scientific and programmatic involvement with the investigators is expected. Oversight is provided at three levels—the NCI program director, a steering committee, and an advisory group. The program director, an extramural scientist administrator of NCI, has substantial authority to assist, guide, coordinate, and participate in the conduct of the Consortium's activities, and also serves as a voting member of the steering committee.

The steering committee, which meets twice a year, is the main governing board of the MMHCC. It sets priorities for model derivation, defines the parameters for model validation, identifies technological impediments to success and strategies for overcoming them, and decides when models should be made available to the cancer research community for individual investigator-initiated projects. Committee voting members include the principal investigator and an additional senior investigator from each U01 or NIH intramural project, the NCI program director, and three members of the NCI Mouse Models Advisory Group. The advisory group consists of NCI and NIH extramural staff who represent the breadth of scientific expertise and program responsibilities that relate to the goals

---

[17] RFA CA-98-013, 1998. See <http://grants.nih.gov/grants/guide/rfa-files/rfa-ca-98-013.html>.

of the MMHCC. It meets regularly to review the progress of the MMHCC, to advise the NCI program director about emerging scientific and technological advances that could further the consortium's goals, and to collaborate on the design and implementation of MMHCC workshops and symposia.

Funding decisions are based on peer review of the scientific merit of applications, in which investigators are asked to address questions regarding the available infrastructure, plans for model derivation, available technology, and plans for interactions with other MMHCC members. The standard review criteria include the significance of the project, the scientific approach, the level of innovation, the qualifications of investigators, and the research environment.

The Consortium was officially launched when 19 groups of investigators from more than 30 institutions were provided with MMHCC funding to develop and evaluate mouse models for cancers of eight major organ systems—breast, prostate, lung, ovary, skin, blood and lymph system, colon, and brain.[18] The Consortium has since grown into an international collaboration involving more than 70 institutions.

Specialized Programs of Research Excellence

In 1992, NCI established the Specialized Programs of Research Excellence (SPOREs)[19] to promote interdisciplinary research through a special $20 million appropriation from Congress. The program focuses on translational research, with the goal of enhancing communication and cooperation between basic and clinical scientists in order to move basic research findings from the laboratory to the clinic more quickly. SPORE scientists are expected to work as teams rather than as independent investigators, with the hope that such collaborations will allow scientists to tackle research questions that could not otherwise be addressed.

SPORE grant applications undergo traditional peer review, but are also assessed on a number of criteria specific to the program. Each proposed research project must be led by co–principal investigators with expertise in basic and clinical research, and must include at least four independent investigators who currently serve as principal investigators on other peer-reviewed research grants. Proposals must also include a minimum of four research projects that represent a "balance and diversity" of translational objectives, such as screening, prevention, diagnosis, and treatment. In addition, NCI requires that a portion of the funds be used to collect and distribute patient tissues and other biological samples.

---

[18] See <http://www.nih.gov/news/pr/dec99/nci-28.htm>.
[19] See <http://spores.nci.nih.gov/>.

SPORE proposals must also include a plan for evaluating the scientific progress and translational potential of all projects, as well as plans for replacing the projects as necessary. This is most often accomplished through annual meetings at which SPORE scientists share data, assess research progress, and identify new research opportunities and priorities. Replacement projects are reviewed by NCI program staff, but do not undergo additional peer review.

SPORE grants are limited to $1.75 million in direct costs and $2.75 million in total costs for 5 years. When first launched, the program solicited grant applications through requests for applications (RFAs), but more recently it has switched to program announcements (PAs) in order to broaden the investigator-initiated applications for all types of cancers (for more information on RFAs and PAs, see Chapter 4). In either case, the P50 funding mechanism (specialized center grant; see Box 4-7 in Chapter 4) has been used to provide grant money through the program.

In 2002, NCI funded SPOREs to study cancers of the breast, prostate, lung, gastrointestinal tract, ovary, genitourinary tract, brain, skin, and head and neck, as well as lymphoma. In the coming years, NCI plans to increase the use of the SPORE mechanism to provide funding for other major cancers, including gynecological tumors, leukemia, myeloma, and pancreatic cancer. However, the report from a recent review of the SPORE program noted that while it is a vital component of NCI's translational research effort, it cannot continue to grow at its present rate. The report also recommended that NCI make a concerted effort to improve the efficiency, effectiveness, and evaluation of SPOREs (National Cancer Advisory Board, 2003).

The Molecular Targets Laboratory

NCI recently awarded a $40 million, 5-year contract to Harvard University to establish a Molecular Targets Laboratory. The goal of this laboratory is to develop research tools, such as protein arrays, and to synthesize thousands of small molecules and screen them for their biological effects (ScienceScope, 2002). Small molecules identified in such screens can provide versatile research tools for the study of protein function (reviewed by Stockwell, 2000) that can be rapidly adopted by many laboratories and also provide the first step toward the development of a new therapeutic drug. The data produced by the Harvard group will form the base for an NCI-sponsored database on chemical genetics. Known as Chembank among some supporters, this database would essentially serve as a chemical version of Genbank, NIH's online repository for genetic data (Adam, 2001a). NCI hopes that scientists from around the world will also deposit their data on the effects of small molecules on proteins, cell pathways, and tissue formation.

The new facility will be an outgrowth of the Harvard Institute of Chemistry and Cell Biology (ICCB),[20] which was founded in 1997 as a collaboration of academic scientists and industrial partners with funding from Merck, Merck KGaA in Germany, and the NCI. The ICCB was established to facilitate collaborations between chemists and cell biologists, and to conduct high-throughput screens of chemical libraries.

RECENT EXAMPLES FROM OTHER BRANCHES OF NIH

The recent doubling of the NIH budget provided new opportunities for the initiation of several large-scale research efforts that might not have been feasible or acceptable to the research community in the past.[21] The relatively large and rapid funding increase allowed NIH to launch new programs even while increasing the number of traditional, investigator-initiated grants (known as R01 grants; see Box 4.7). This phenomenon is perhaps most striking for the National Institute of General Medical Sciences (NIGMS), traditionally known as the "R01 Institute," which established several new large-scale initiatives in recent years, several of which are described below. A program established by the National Institute for Allergy and Infectious Diseases for distributing tools and reagents made possible by large-scale genomics projects is also described.

NIGMS Glue Grants

NIGMS launched a new initiative to fund large-scale collaborative projects in 1999. This initiative was the result of consultations with leaders in the scientific community who said that the most challenging biological problems require the expertise and input of large, multifaceted groups of scientists. The projects are referred to as "glue grants" because they are meant to provide the resources necessary to bring scientists together to focus on a research topic, with the goal of addressing problems beyond the reach of individual investigators.

An RFA was issued in 1999,[22] with the expectation that participating investigators would already hold funded research grants related to a proposed topic of study that was of central importance to biomedical science and to the mission of NIGMS. Support for new individual research projects was not the intent of these large-scale project awards; rather, a signifi-

---

[20] See <http://sbweb.med.harvard.edu/~iccb/>.

[21] Judith Greenberg, acting director of NIGMS, in a presentation to the National Cancer Policy Board on July 16, 2002.

[22] RFA GM-99-007, May 26, 1999. See <http://grants.nih.gov/grants/guide/rfa-files/RFA-GM-99-007.html>.

cant level of support was offered so that investigators could extend their research efforts by forming a consortium to approach a research problem of overarching importance in a comprehensive and highly integrated fashion. It was noted in the RFA that:

> Biomedical science has entered a new era where these collaborations are becoming critical to rapid progress. This is the result of several factors. First, not every laboratory has the breadth to pursue problems that increasingly must be solved through the application of a multitude of approaches. These include the involvement of fields such as physics, engineering, mathematics, and computer science that were previously considered peripheral to mainstream biomedical science. Second, the ability to attack large projects that involve considerable data collection and technology development requires the collaboration of many groups and laboratories. Finally, large-scale, expensive technologies such as combinatorial chemistry, DNA chips, high throughput mass spectrometric analysis, etc., are not readily available to all laboratories that could benefit from their use. These technologies require specialized expertise, but could lend themselves to management by specialists who collaborate or offer services to others.

In the fall of 2000, NIGMS announced that it would provide $5 million for the first year to a consortium of basic scientists called the Alliance for Cellular Signaling (AFCS), with the expectation of spending a projected total of $25 million on the project over the course of 5 years.[23] The project aims to study all aspects of cellular communication in two cell types: cardiomyocytes and B-cells. The primary goal of the effort is to map the immense complexity of intracellular signals in both cell types, with the ultimate objective of being able to search for and test "in silico"[24] new therapeutic compounds that affect these signaling pathways.

The AFCS is a consortium of approximately 50 scientists working at 20 different academic institutions around the country. AFCS investigators work in core laboratories located at several different academic centers, including the California Institute of Technology in Pasadena; the San Francisco Veterans Administration Medical Center; Stanford University; the University of California, San Diego; and University of Texas Southwestern. Two biotechnology companies will also participate in AFCS studies by providing custom-made materials, such as antisense reagents (ISIS Pharmaceuticals of Carlsbad, California) and two-hybrid analysis technology, a method used to track interactions between proteins inside cells (Myriad Genetics, Inc., of Salt Lake City, Utah).

---

[23] NIH News release, September 5, 2001. See <http://www.nigms.nih.gov/funding/gluegrant_release.html>.

[24] Using a computer model rather than traditional laboratory experiments.

All of the data produced in the core laboratories will be deposited immediately in a publicly accessible database, and investigators will relinquish patent rights to the information. Once the data have been posted publicly, any scientist, whether a member of the AFCS or not, can use them for research that may lead to patents. The consortium also uses virtual conferencing via the Internet2, a university-based version of the Internet, to encourage open and rapid communication among members.

In addition to support from NIGMS, other funding for the AFCS project will be provided by several nonprofit organizations and pharmaceutical companies. They include Eli Lilly and Company, Johnson and Johnson, the Merck Genome Research Institute, Novartis Pharmaceuticals Corporation, Chiron Therapeutics, Aventis, and the Agouron Institute.

In the fall of 2001, NIGMS announced the provision of $8 million for a second glue grant to the Cell Migration Consortium. The institute plans to spend an estimated $38 million on the project over the next 5 years. The project will bring together a large group of disparate scientists (biologists, chemists, biophysicists, optical physicists, mathematicians, computer scientists, geneticists, and engineers) from 12 academic medical centers across the country to study the mechanism of how cells move. A secondary goal of the Consortium is to facilitate the translation of new discoveries in cell migration into the development of novel therapeutic drugs and treatments. Understanding of cell migration could potentially lead to advances against a variety of diseases, such as cancer, in which cell movement leads to lethal metastases. Two additional glue grants have since been awarded for a study of Inflammation and the Host Response to Injury and for a Consortium for Functional Glycomics.

The selection of proposed consortia for funding is based on traditional NIH peer review. The standard review criteria are used, including the significance of the proposed project, the experimental approach, the degree of innovation, the qualifications of investigators, and the scientific environment. Applications are actually made in two phases. Phase I applicants submit an overview of the proposed large-scale project for peer review. The purpose of this first phase is to provide resources for detailed planning to applicants who have demonstrated the selection of an appropriate complex biological problem, an innovative plan, and appropriate commitments to its solution from participating investigators and institutions. Successful Phase I applicants receive a $25,000 planning grant, and those applicants who receive awards are eligible to submit a more extensively planned and detailed application for a Phase II award to support the large-scale project itself. Phase II applications must provide specific intermediate goals (milestones) and a timeline for their accomplishment. These goals are adjusted annually at the award anniversary date to incorporate accomplishments made to date, progress in the field, and input from an advisory committee. Applications must also include an administrative management plan, a project management plan, and a plan for data sharing and intellectual property.

In addition to the principal investigator and participating investigators, other essential components of a large-scale collaborative project include a steering committee, an external advisory committee, and a program director. The steering committee is largely responsible for governance of the project and plays a major role in developing goals and operating procedures. The committee is chaired by the principal investigator, and its membership is chosen from participating investigators and project staff. The external advisory committee meets annually with the steering committee to assess progress and provide feedback on proposed goals for the next year of support. The members of this committee, who are not involved in the project, are appointed by the principal investigator in consultation with the steering committee and with the approval of the NIGMS program director after the Phase II award has been made. The NIGMS program director has considerable influence over the project by facilitating interactions between the steering and advisory committees and by facilitating communication with the scientific community directly affected by the collaborative project. The program director also serves as a voting member of the steering committee.

The RFA for large-scale collaborative projects was reannounced in 2001.[25] In addition, a related PA was published in 2000. Entitled "Integrative and Collaborative Approaches to Research,"[26] the purpose of this initiative is to provide groups of currently funded investigators at different institutions with additional support for collaborative and integrative activities. The initiative is intended to support collaborative research and resources on a modest scale, involving a small number of funded investigators working on a common problem. The maximum direct cost per year is $300,000. Unlike an RFA, a PA is an ongoing announcement for which there is no set-aside of funds.

NIGMS Protein Structure Initiative

NIGMS recently launched a new large-scale, cooperative effort known as the Protein Structure Initiative (PSI) (Smaglik, 2000). The goal of the 10-

---

[25] RFA GM-01-004, February 28, 2001. See <http://grants.nih.gov/grants/guide/rfa-files/RFA-GM-01-004.html>.

[26] PA-00-099, May 24, 2000. See <http://grants.nih.gov/grants/guide/pa-files/PA-00-099.html>.

year project is to foster the new field of structural genomics.[27] Following the completion of the human and other genome projects, a crucial next step in understanding biology is determining the structure and function of the entire set of gene products (Burley, 2000). Sequences from the human genome are being analyzed to identify distinct protein families. Structural genomics uses these computational analyses, along with structural determinations of the protein products, to advance the study of protein function.

The project will take place in two distinct stages. The first 5 years will be focused on technology development, while the remaining 5 years will be devoted to determining the structures of proteins in various protein families from different organisms, including bacteria, yeast, roundworms, fruit flies, and humans. In September 2001, NIGMS awarded almost $30 million to seven research centers, each receiving approximately $4 million for the first year. The Institute anticipates spending a total of around $150 million on these projects over 5 years. The projects at the research centers are intended to serve as pilots leading to subsequent large-scale research networks in structural genomics. The first goal is to improve and automate methodologies for X-ray crystallography and magnetic resonance spectroscopy. Although structure determination techniques have advanced dramatically in recent years, they are still time-consuming and labor-intensive. The centers are attempting to speed up and decrease the cost of every aspect of the process: protein family classification and target selection, protein expression, protein purification, sample preparation (crystallization or isotopic labeling), structure determination, and analyses of results. The effort to develop high-throughput technologies will require the skills of chemists, engineers, and computer scientists, as well as biologists. Unlike the field of genomics, which was accelerated by robotic DNA sequencers, structural biology and proteomics are unlikely to be dominated by a single technology (Service, 2001c). Moreover, a recent International Conference on Structural Genomics revealed that technology development is complex and unpredictable (Service, 2002).

The second 5-year phase was intended to focus on full-scale production. The plan was to organize all known proteins into structural families based on their genetic sequences. The goal was then to determine the structure of a few proteins from each family, for a total of about 10,000 protein structures by the end of 10 years. However, the current pace of the effort suggests that this goal is unlikely to be achieved in the expected timeframe, so NIGMS will need to make difficult decisions about how to proceed for the second 5 years (Service, 2002). The information generated

---

[27] NIH news release, September 26, 2000; see <http://www.nigms.nih.gov/news/releases/ SGpilots.html>.

in the second phase is intended to form the foundation of a public resource linking sequence, structural, and functional information. This resource could also allow scientists to use gene sequences to predict the approximate structures of other proteins.

There is also much interest among pharmaceutical and biotechnology companies in pursuing structural genomics projects (Smaglik, 2000, Service, 2001a-c). However, industry researchers are more likely to focus on medically relevant proteins, rather than whole classes of proteins. Moreover, companies are often more interested in the structures of proteins with different compounds bound to them than in the structure of the protein alone. The public project, in contrast, seeks breadth of basic data through the selection of proteins covering a wide variety of structures. The main goal of the NIGMS-sponsored project is to develop a detailed database that can serve as a valuable resource and research tool for scientists engaged in both basic and clinically relevant research. In this regard, the project is quite similar to the publicly funded HGP. Nonetheless, some public–private collaborations in structural genomics have also been initiated (Stevens et al., 2001; Service, 2002). For example, the NIGMS-funded Joint Center for Structural Genomics (JCSG) has contracted work with the Genomics Institute of the Novartis Research Foundation, which is collaborating with biotechnology companies like Syrrx to speed technology development. The JCSG is also seeking collaborations with international structural genomics consortia to improve high-throughput technologies. Such consortia have been launched in many countries, including Japan, Great Britain, and Canada, in the last 2 years (Stevens et al., 2001).

The NIGMS-funded PSI encompasses two PAs[28] and an RFA. (For more information on the PA and RFA funding mechanisms, see Chapter 4). These announcements resulted in part from recommendations made at three NIGMS-sponsored workshops focused on structural genomics, held in 1998 and 1999. The RFA[29] was issued in 1999 and again in 2000, but will not be reissued. The seven awards described above, plus two more awarded in the second round, were made through the RFA. The two PAs encourage scientists to develop new methods and technologies for enhancing the efficiency of structure determination by developing high-throughput approaches. The PAs are ongoing and provide support for traditional individual research grants (R01), program projects (P01), and small-business research grants (Small Business Innovation Research [SBIR]/Small Business Technology Transfer [STTR]).

In the case of grants made through the RFA (using the P50 research center award mechanism), NIH has set forth a number of special require-

---

[28] PA-99-117 June 25, 1999; PA-99-116 June 25, 1999.
[29] RFA GM-99-009, June 3, 1999; RFA GM-00-006, July 24, 2000 (Re-announcement).

ments for application and post award management. Applicants are solely responsible for the planning, direction, and execution of their projects, so effective plans for management and administration of the research center are crucial for the application process. The principal investigator is expected to make any adjustments in scientific direction necessary to accommodate the continually changing technological environment. Each research center must appoint its own external scientific advisory committee, composed of research scientists not involved in the consortium, to provide independent assessment and advice to the principal investigator and staff. This committee is expected to meet at least twice each year. Significant changes in project direction must be reported to NIGMS staff, and scientific and programmatic visits to the grantee are conducted to ensure that the project remains focused on appropriate goals, incorporates new technological advances, and makes sufficient progress. The benchmarks used to assess progress may be changed annually, and NIGMS may include outside consultants in the annual progress review. Funds may be reduced or withheld for failure to meet milestones agreed upon by grantees and NIH staff. In addition, grant recipients are also required to attend annual meetings at NIH to discuss progress and results.

Grant applicants must also present plans for adherence to several policies adopted by NIGMS regarding research training, intellectual property, and data release. Because the research projects of the PSI involve extensive data collection and technology development with limited hypothesis-driven aspects, NIGMS generally considers them inappropriate as research training projects for graduate students and postdoctoral scientists. The work is more likely to require project managers and technicians. Thus, applicants planning to employ graduate students or postdoctoral fellows on their project must justify the request.

NIGMS monitors its grant recipients' activities with respect to patenting the structural results and technology developments as well. The results of the structural genomics projects are meant to be freely available for use by the entire research community, and therefore must be deposited promptly,[30] prior to publication, in the Protein Data Bank (PDB),

---

[30] According to the NIGMS Statement on Coordinate Deposition for Structural Genomics, an international agreement called for releasing structure information on most proteins soon after completion, but setting aside some structures for a limited period of time (less than 6 months) to allow for application for patents. Because the NIH research centers are just beginning their work, it is unclear how much time is needed to ensure that the results are accurate and to prepare the results for publication and deposition in the Protein Data Bank. The current goal of the PSI is to limit this time to 4 to 6 weeks. This should also be adequate time for the investigators to file patent applications for protein structures of commercial interest. See <http://www.nigms.nih.gov/funding/psi.html> [accessed 9/24/01].

which is in the public domain. Grantees are also required to develop and maintain their own public website containing information on strategies for target selection, the status of research on these proteins, technological and methodology findings, high-throughput approaches, efficiency, and cost analyses.

The Pathogen Functional Genomics Resource Center

The National Institute of Allergy and Infectious Diseases (NIAID) recently established a centralized facility providing the research community with resources for conducting functional genomics research on human pathogens and invertebrate vectors.[31] NIAID awarded a 5-year, $25 million contract to TIGR to establish the Pathogen Functional Genomics Resource Center (PFGRC), which will provide scientists with microarrays, gene clones, and other reagents and tools for genomics research (Malakoff, 2001). A scientific advisory committee provides advice to NIAID to assist in guiding the activities of the PFGRC. The impetus for the new center was in part to avoid funding duplicate requests to NIAID by centralizing some toolmaking and training activities, but the center can also now make standardized research tools more easily available to microbial researchers, including those at small institutions who would not otherwise have such access. The Institute plans to select ten organisms for reagent development in the next 3 years, three of which are being developed for the first year.[32] The PFGRC also aims to support the development of emerging genomic technologies and to train scientists in the latest techniques in functional genomics.

Because the microarrays are limited in quantity, scientists interested in obtaining them must submit brief proposals to NIAID describing research plans for their utilization. The microarrays will be provided (150 slides for a given organism per request) for both exploratory/developmental and established research projects. Proposals, limited to five pages, must include a research plan stating the specific aims, the significance of the research question, the potential impact on the field, and the experimental design to be used. Applicants must also provide documentation that they have access to the resources and expertise necessary to design, perform, and interpret the experiments, including data analysis. In addition, requestors must agree to NIAID's data release policy, which requires the timely dissemination of microarray data in either a publicly developed database supported by the PFGRC or another publicly available

---

[31] See <http://www.niaid.nih.gov/dmid/genomes/pfgrc/>.

[32] Further details about how organisms are selected can be found at <http://pfgrc.tigr.org>.

database, as designated by NIAID. Requests are reviewed in a confidential manner by a committee following the usual NIH peer review criteria (significance, approach, investigator, and environment). Investigators are selected on the overall merit of the proposal, but the availability of reagents may also be taken into consideration. NIAID anticipates that the review process can be completed within 2 weeks of the deadline for receipt of applications.

The Women's Health Initiative

The NIH launched the Women's Health Initiative (WHI) in 1991 with the broad goal of investigating strategies for the prevention and control of some of the most common causes of morbidity and mortality among postmenopausal women, including cancer, cardiovascular disease, and osteoporotic fractures.[33] In October 1997, the WHI was transferred to the National Heart, Lung, and Blood Institute (NHLBI), where it has functioned as a consortium effort led by NHLBI in cooperation with NCI and the National Institute of Arthritis and Musculoskeletal and Skin Diseases.

The WHI is one of the largest studies of its kind ever undertaken in the United States (see Table 3-1). The effects of hormone replacement therapy (HRT) and diet on the health of postmenopausal women were investigated for almost a decade prior to the WHI. Because of a lack of funds, however, no studies of sufficient size and duration to test with confidence the value and risks of these approaches had been initiated (Rossouw et al., 1995). The WHI involves more than 40 centers nationwide and 162,000 women aged 50–79, about 18 percent of whom represent minority groups. Enrollment in the study began in 1993 and ended in 1998. Participants will be followed for 8 to 12 years.

The WHI consists of three studies:

- A *clinical trial* that tests the effects of three different prevention approaches—HRT, diet modification, and calcium and vitamin D supplementation—on heart disease, cancer risk, and osteoporosis. All three approaches are being studied using a randomized, controlled trial design. Depending on their eligibility, women chose to enroll in one, two, or all three parts of the clinical study. Altogether, the three components involve 68,000 women who are randomized to receive the different interventions.

- An *observational study* involving about 94,000 women to investigate the interplay among health, lifestyle, and other disease risk factors. The goal is to identify predictors and biological markers for disease. The

---

[33] See <http://www.nhlbi.nih.gov/health/public/heart/other/whi/wmn_hlt.htm>.

TABLE 3-1   Women's Health Initiative Costs

Clinical Trial and Observational Study Budget	Average Cost per Year (in millions of dollars)	Total Cost All Years (~15 years) (in millions of dollars)
Clinical Coordinating Center	11.7	175.5
40 Clinical Centers	35.3	530.0
Total	**47.0**	**705.5**
Clinical Trial by Component		
Calcium, Vitamin D	1.2	18.2
Hormone Replacement Therapy	15.5	232.4
Dietary Modification	27.7	415.1
Observational Study	2.6	39.8
Total	**47.0**	**705.5**

Clinical and Observational Study Cost per Participant	Number Enrolled	Average Cost per Year (in dollars)	Total Cost All Years (in dollars)
Observational Study	93,676	28	425
Calcium/Vitamin D	36,282	33	501
Hormone Replacement Therapy	27,347	567	8499
Dietary Modification	48,836	567	8499
All Clinical Trials and Observational Studies	161,809*	291	4360

Community Prevention Study	Total Cost (in millions of dollars)
1994	0.16
1995	4.0
1996	4.0
1997	4.0
1998	4.2
1999	4.0
Total	**20.36**

Women's Health Initiative	Total Cost (in millions of dollars)
	725.8

*Because some participants may be enrolled in more than one study or trial at the same time, this number represents the total number of enrolled participants, but is not a sum of the numbers above it.

SOURCE: Personal communication with Jacques Rossouw, director, Women's Health Initiative, Office of the Director, NHLBI, March 2002.

women receive no specific intervention, but their medical history and health habits are followed over the course of the study.

• A *community prevention study* to determine how women can best be encouraged to adopt healthful behaviors, such as an improved eating plan, nutritional supplementation, smoking cessation, physical activity, and early detection of treatable health problems. Conducted through eight community prevention centers based at universities, the 5-year study is aimed at developing model programs that can be implemented nationwide. This study entails a unique 5-year cooperative venture with CDC.

The Fred Hutchinson Cancer Research Center in Seattle, Washington, serves as the WHI Clinical Coordinating Center for data collection, management, and analysis. The WHI is a large-scale-science project not so much because it is employing high technology to discover biological processes, but more because of its size and collaborative nature. The initiative is focused on studying the impact of practical and feasible interventions for diseases common among women by involving hundreds of investigators at scores of institutions, at a cost of hundred of millions of dollars.

Surprising findings were recently reported for the WHI's HRT trial, and that portion of the study was terminated 3 years early for ethical reasons on the basis of those results (Rossouw et al., 2002; Enserink, 2002b). Although many previous observational studies had indicated that HRT was beneficial for reducing cardiovascular disease, the randomized, controlled trial of the WHI showed an increase in heart disease, stroke, and pulmonary embolisms, as well as an increase in invasive breast cancer, among women taking estrogen and progesterone. Although HRT reduced the incidence of bone fractures and colorectal cancer, these benefits did not outweigh the other risks. A similar large-scale study of HRT in the United Kingdom[34] was also halted as a result of the apparent risks identified by the WHI study, despite criticism of the design and analysis of the U.S. study (Enserink, 2002a; Couzin and Enserink, 2002).

VACCINE RESEARCH

A large-scale approach to research is becoming the norm in the field of vaccine development, especially with respect to AIDS (acquired immune deficiency) vaccine research. The field has been boosted by a large influx of funding in recent years from both federal and philanthropic sources. The Bill and Melinda Gates Foundation has provided more than $125 million for the International AIDS Vaccine Initiative since its cre-

---

[34] Women's International Study of Long Duration Oestrogen After Menopause (Wisdom).

ation in 1999 (Cohen, 2002), and NIH has made a similar investment in targeted research for vaccine research in the United States.

In May 1997, President Clinton set a goal to develop an AIDS vaccine within 10 years. NIH responded by creating the Vaccine Research Center (VRC),[35] a state-of-the-art biomedical research laboratory to facilitate multidisciplinary research aimed at vaccine development. Although the primary focus of VRC research is the development of an AIDS vaccine, the center also has a broader mission to advance the development of vaccines for all diseases, based on the premise that what is learned with other diseases may be helpful in the research on AIDS, and vice versa. The center focuses primarily on the preclinical and early clinical stages of vaccine development, but works closely with the HIV Vaccine Trials Network, which conducts all phases of clinical trials.

A novel venture within the NIH intramural research program, the VRC receives joint funding from NIAID and NCI and is spearheaded by NIAID, NCI, and the NIH Office of AIDS Research. A new building for the center, costing between $35–40 million, officially opened in spring 2001. The center had an operating budget of $26 million for fiscal year 2000, but the budget has increased as the program has expanded to full capacity. The center employs about 100 scientists and support staff, including tenure-track scientists, staff scientists, postdoctoral fellows, and graduate students, drawn from an array of disciplines such as immunology, virology, and vaccine development (Gershon, 2000). The VCR also works with scientists in academic, clinical, and industrial laboratories through a program of national and international collaborations. In addition, the VRC is directed to actively seek industrial partners for the development, efficacy testing, and marketing of vaccines.

NATIONAL SCIENCE FOUNDATION'S SCIENCE AND TECHNOLOGY CENTERS PROGRAM

The Science and Technology Centers (STC) Program of the National Science Foundation (NSF) was established in 1987 to fund basic research and education activities and to encourage technology transfer and innovative approaches to interdisciplinary programs.[36] The program offered a novel approach to research by creating large, multidisciplinary programs at universities. STC grants, which are open to researchers working in any area typically supported by NSF, provide up to $20 million over 5 years, with a possibility for 5 additional years of support pending the results of an exten-

---

[35] See <http://www.niaid.nih.gov/vrc/default.htm>.
[36] See <http://www.nsf.gov/od/oia/programs/stc/start.htm>.

sive midterm review. The program thus provides a mechanism by which the basic research community can take a relatively long-term view of science.

The goals of the STC Program are to enable academic research teams to:

• Exploit opportunities in science and engineering in which the complexity of the research problems or the resources needed to solve them require the advantages of collaborative relationships that can best be provided by campus-based research centers.
• Involve students, research scientists, and engineers in partnerships to enhance the training and employability of professionals through an awareness of potential applications for scientific discoveries.
• Provide long-term, stable funding at a level that encourages risk taking and ensures a solid foundation for attracting quality undergraduate and graduate students (with special emphasis on women and minorities) into science and technology careers.
• Facilitate the transfer of knowledge among academia, industry, and national laboratories.

Thus STCs are expected not only to serve as critical national resources for research, but also to improve education in local schools; strengthen undergraduate and graduate training; improve minority representation in the sciences; and develop collaborations with other academic institutions, industry, and the community.

There have been four competitions for STC grants, with the first centers being funded in 1989. Six new centers were selected in 2002, bringing the total number of STC awards to date to 36. Only 2 centers have been terminated for falling short of their stated goals. Selection entails a 2-year process of proposal development, review, revision, and site visits, with a proposal's management plan being key to an applicant's success. Funding is provided through cooperative agreements with NSF and comes with extensive hands-on supervision by NSF officials (Mervis, 2002).

Initially, the program was controversial.[37] Scientists worried that the proposed centers would drain funds from NSF's traditional support for individual investigators, or that they would promote applied research at the expense of basic science (Mervis, 2002). However, the program's annual budget of $45 million is only 1.1 percent of NSF's overall research budget, and many centers focus on very basic research. Indeed, agency officials report that many countries have sought NSF's advice in creating similar programs (Mervis, 2002). Furthermore, a 1996 review of the program by the NRC was quite positive. The review panel concluded:

---

[37] The program likely would have been even more controversial if many issues had not already been addressed in the late 1970s in establishing the Engineering Research Centers, which were NSF's first large-scale multidisciplinary centers in universities.

Most STCs are producing high-quality world-class research that would not have been possible without a center structure and presence. . . . The design of the STC program has produced an effective means for identifying particularly important scientific problems that require a center mode of support. Many STCs also provide a model for the creative interaction of scientists, engineers, and students in various disciplines and across academic, industry, and other institutional boundaries (NRC, 1996: page 2).

The panel also suggested that the center approach was a valuable and necessary tool in NSF's portfolio of support mechanisms, and that the nation and NSF were getting a good return on their relatively small investment. One program cited in the report as particularly successful was the Center for Biological Timing. The panel noted that this center had produced an impressive scholarly output in terms of both quantity and quality, and that these studies could realistically have been accomplished only through center support because of their complexity and long-term nature, as well as the unlikelihood of their being supported through traditional investigator-initiated programs. Indeed, the panel concluded in general that the STC mode of support allows certain types of research problems to be addressed that otherwise would not be taken up. The panel noted that research problems fall along a spectrum—some being well suited to an individual-investigator approach to inquiry, others to a center mode, and still others to a facility model—with STCs serving as one means of support that helps balance the NSF portfolio of funding instruments.

Thus, the NRC panel recommended that NSF continue the STC program. A number of additional recommendations for improving the program included placing greater weight on scientific and administrative leadership in evaluating proposals for STCs and in the periodic reviews of centers (NRC, 1996). Two other independent reviews at about the same time came to similarly positive conclusions, and also resulted in recommendations for improving administration and oversight of the program (NAPA, 1995; ABT Associates, 1996).

THE SNP CONSORTIUM

Single nucleotide polymorphisms, or SNPs, are common, small variations that occur in human DNA throughout the genome. These polymorphic markers can be used to map and identify important genes associated with diseases, and thereby provide a valuable resource for taking the first step in developing new diagnostic tests or therapies. They can also be responsible themselves for genetic differences that predispose some individuals to disease and that underlie variability in individual responses to treatment.

The potential value of SNPs generated great interest in both the public and private sectors in identifying and mapping a large number of polymorphic markers, and discussions about establishing a public–private consortium to undertake such a project began in 1998. This type of cooperative arrangement may appear to be at odds with the business goals of private companies, but it was widely recognized that the industry would be better off if information on SNPs were made freely available to all, without the restrictions that could develop if many different organizations held patents on markers scattered throughout the genome. Through collaboration, a high-density, high-quality map could be created more quickly, and with shared financial risk and less duplication of effort than if each company pursued development of a SNP map on its own. These discussions led to the establishment of the SNP Consortium in 1999.

The SNP Consortium[38] is a nonprofit entity comprising the Wellcome Trust and a group of pharmaceutical and technical companies.[39] Its mission is to identify SNPs distributed evenly throughout the human genome and to make information on these SNPs available to the public without intellectual property restrictions. It is governed by a board composed of representatives of the member organizations and led by an independent chairman. The consortium participants provide oversight and technical expertise for the project, and also direct the effort to ensure the public availability of the SNPs that are generated. The consortium files patent applications, but with the declared policy of later abandoning them or converting them to a statutory registration of invention, which simply precludes others from patenting the discovery. Confirmed SNPs have been placed in the public domain at quarterly intervals as they have become available, thus providing free and equal access to all in the worldwide medical research community.

---

[38] See <http://snp.cshl.org/index.html>.

[39] In addition to the Wellcome Trust, the SNP encompasses 13 pharmaceutical and technical companies: APBiotech, AstraZeneca PLC, Aventis Pharma, Bayer AG, Bristol-Myers Squibb Company, F. Hoffman-La Roche, Glaxo Wellcome PLC, IBM, Motorola, Novartis Pharmaceuticals, Pfizer Inc, Searle, and SmithKline Beecham PLC. The work supported by the consortium is performed at four major centers for molecular genetics: the Whitehead Institute for Biomedical Research, Washington University School of Medicine in St. Louis, the Wellcome Trust's Sanger Centre, and the Stanford Human Genome Center. The Cold Spring Harbor Laboratory maintains the consortium's databases. Orchid BioSciences, Inc., performs third-party validation and quality control testing on SNPs identified through the consortium's research.

Recently, the SNP Consortium collaborated with the International Human Genome Sequencing Consortium[40] to publish a paper in the journal *Nature* describing a map of 1.42 million validated SNPs distributed throughout the human genome (Sachidanandam et al., 2001). Using DNA from a diversified, representative panel of anonymous volunteers, the collaborators identified, on average, one SNP for every 1.9 kilobases of DNA. Such collaboration further demonstrates that public–private cooperation can be an efficient means of developing basic research tools.

In the case of SNP analysis, however, international cooperation was perhaps not as strong as it had been for the Human Genome Project. The SNP Consortium invited Japanese companies to participate in the project, but they declined the offer. Instead, 40 Japanese drug firms decided to provide a total of $10 million to university researchers in Japan to study SNPs in that country's population. They will establish their own database of SNPs, but these data will also be made freely available to other scientists (Sciencescope, 2000).

A new public–private consortium was recently established to further build on the work of both the SNP Consortium and the HGP. The $100 million HapMap project, with funds from six countries[41] and several pharmaceutical companies, aims to map about 300,000 haplotypes from four populations in Africa, Asia, and the United States within 3 years (Couzin, 2002b; Adam, 2001b). Haplotypes are sets of genetic markers that are close enough on a particular chromosome to be inherited together. Using SNPs alone to identify disease-associated genes can be difficult and expensive, partly because it is difficult to trace individual SNPs in a genome containing 3 billion base pairs. Haplotype analysis will reduce background noise and should make the search for genes easier and faster because the many individual markers are consolidated into more manageable clusters.

Scientists realized only recently that a haplotype map might be feasible when they discovered that relatively large blocks of DNA are inherited in this way. Computer simulations predicted that DNA haplotypes

---

[40] This collaborative effort was funded by the National Human Genome Research Institute and the SNP Consortium. Three academic genome research centers—the Whitehead Institute for Biomedical Research in Cambridge, Massachusetts; Washington University School of Medicine in St. Louis; and the Sanger Centre in Hinxton, United Kingdom—participated directly in this collaboration. The International Human Genome Sequencing Consortium includes scientists at 16 institutions in France, Germany, Japan, China, Great Britain, and the United States, with funding from government agencies and public charities in several countries.

[41] Funders include NIH in the United States ($40 million) and the Wellcome Trust in the United Kingdom ($25 million).

would only be about 10,000 or fewer bases. To their surprise, genome researchers have found that haplotype blocks tend to be much larger (up to 100,000 base pairs), and that many such blocks come in just a few different versions. For example, within some sequence stretches of 50,000 bases, only four of five patterns of SNPs, or haplotypes, might account for 80–90 percent of the population. It is not clear why this occurs, but some chromosome regions may be less likely than others to recombine during meiosis, leading to conservation of the DNA blocks (Helmuth, 2001).

Haplotypes are found by analyzing genotype data, so the new collaboration will essentially be a high-throughput genotyping effort. The work will be done by several biotechnology companies and public laboratories, including the Sanger Center and the Whitehead Institute, but decisions are still pending on such issues as how data collection will be standardized, how the map will be structured, and how the work will be divided. It is hoped that the new map will provide an invaluable tool to simplify the search for associations between DNA variations and complex diseases such as cancer, diabetes, and mental illness. However, many scientists, especially population geneticists, have questioned the value of generating a haplotype map at this time, arguing that there is too little information on the usefulness of such a map or how to best to proceed (Couzin, 2002a).

There is also great interest in developing more efficient, cost-effective technologies for high-throughput analysis of SNPs (Chicurel, 2001). Without such improvements, screening large populations to search for disease- or therapy-associated genes could still be impractical. A number of investigators are attempting to improve on the current technology, but to date no coordinated effort has been made.

HUMAN PROTEOME ORGANIZATION

The Human Proteome Organization (HUPO) is an international alliance of industry, academic, and government scientists aimed at determining the structure and function of all proteins made by the human body (Kaiser, 2002; Abbott, 2001). The mission[42] of HUPO is threefold: to consolidate national and regional proteome organizations; to engage in scientific and educational activities that encourage the spread of proteomics technologies, as well as the free dissemination of knowledge pertaining to the human proteome and that of model organisms; and to assist in the coordination of public proteome initiatives. The organization's formation was spurred by concerns that in the absence of such a coordinated effort,

---

[42] http://www.hupo.org/.

> **BOX 3-2 Five Initial Proposed Projects of the
> Human Proteome Organization**
>
> **Plasma proteome:** Identify less-abundant proteins in blood, initially in healthy adults.
> **Antibody Initiative:** Build a library of antibodies for 30,000 gene products.
> **Cell Models:** Carry out a liver proteome project; coordinate data standards for heart
> and other existing proteome studies.
> **Bioinformatics:** Develop databases, analysis software, and annotation standards.
> **New Technology:** Develop methods for quantifying 5,000 proteins and their interac-
> tions in a tissue or cell type.
>
> ―――――――――
>
> SOURCE: Kaiser (2002).

individual companies would generate their own basic proteomics data and protect them through trade secrecy. The organizers hope to include more countries than participated in the HGP, and plan to generate funding contributions from companies, with matching government funds.

HUPO participants have proposed five initial research and technology development projects to garner interest from potential funders (see Box 3-2). Several companies have already offered financial support, and a number of countries are launching initiatives related to HUPO's goals. The NIGMS Alliance for Cellular Signaling is one such initiative, but a broader role for NIH in a global proteomics project remains unclear. Some U.S. proteomics experts have proposed establishing a few pilot large-scale centers to identify proteins en masse with uniform standards from healthy and diseased tissues and blood serum (Kaiser, 2002). But many others question the sensitivity and specificity of current mass spectrometers, suggesting that such an undertaking would be premature, and that it would be more useful to fund individual investigators to study small parts of large, complex protein networks (Check, 2002).

HOWARD HUGHES MEDICAL INSTITUTE

The Howard Hughes Medical Institute (HHMI) provides an example of an alternative strategy that could be used to undertake large-scale research projects. HHMI is a nonprofit medical research organization that employs more than 300 biomedical scientists across the United States at more than 70 universities, medical centers, and other research organizations. It also maintains a grants program aimed at enhancing science education at all levels. One of the world's largest philanthropies, HHMI had an endowment in mid-2000 of approximately $13 billion, and $600 million was disbursed for medical research ($466 million), science education, and related activities.

Created by Hughes in 1953, the Institute has always been committed to basic research, with the charge of probing "the genesis of life itself."[43] The organization's charter states that "the primary purpose and objective of the Howard Hughes Medical Institute shall be the promotion of human knowledge within the field of the basic sciences (principally the field of medical research and medical education) and the effective application thereof for the benefit of mankind." The Institute draws a clear distinction between itself and other foundations that provide money for biomedical research in that it operates as an organization with investigators across the country. Hughes investigators are employed by the Institute but conduct their research in the laboratories of their host institutions. The Institute's work has traditionally focused on five main areas of research: cell biology, genetics, immunology, neuroscience, and structural biology. More recently, clinical science programs have been added, as well as a new focus on bioinformatics. Investigators are free to pursue their own research interests without the burden of writing detailed proposals for each project, but their research progress is reviewed by HHMI every 5 years. Scientists who are not renewed as HHMI investigators are provided with additional phase-out funds for 2–3 years so they will have an opportunity to seek other funds or gradually scale back their activities. This approach also eases the strain on affected staff and trainees in the lab who need time to seek other positions.

In what was perhaps the Institute's first foray into large-scale science (as defined in this report), HHMI held an Informational Forum on the Human Genome at NIH in 1986. Subsequently, HHMI played a role in the HGP by supporting several databases, including one at Yale University; one at the Centre D'Etude du Polymorphisme Humaine in Paris; and one at the Jackson Laboratory in Bar Harbor, Maine (Cook-Deegan, 1994).

Recently, HHMI announced a novel research endeavor for the organization. This new 10-year, $500 million project[44] may be viewed as another form of large-scale science funded by a nonprofit organization. HHMI plans to build a permanent biomedical research center that will develop advanced technology for biomedical scientists and provide a collaborative setting for the development of new research tools. Slated to open in 2005, the new center will have an annual operating budget of about $50 million (Kaiser, 2001). Research topics have not yet been fully defined, but are likely to focus on such areas as bioinformatics, proteomics, and imag-

---

[43] http://www.hhmi.org/.
[44] See <http://www.hhmi.org/news/020101.html>.

ing tools (e.g., electron microscopy). Investigators are likely to include computational scientists, chemists, physicists, engineers, and biomedical scientists with cross-disciplinary expertise.

The center will provide laboratories for up to 24 investigators (who will not have tenure), plus their research staffs, for a total of 200–300 people. In addition, laboratories and other facilities will be built for visiting researchers and core scientific support resources. Visiting scientists will be able to stay for as little as a few weeks or may take a sabbatical year. Organizers hope this format will allow for rapid shifts into new areas that show unusual scientific promise and for quick adaptation of new discoveries for use in biological research and health-related sciences.

For collaborative research at the new center, HHMI will request proposals from the scientific community at large, as well as from its own investigators. The Institute will seek out proposals focused on cutting-edge scientific and technological goals, and will give preference to projects that bring together diverse individuals and expertise from different environments. To be successful, proposals will have to demonstrate originality, creativity, and a high degree of scientific risk taking. One goal of these collaborations is to ensure that all HHMI investigators, regardless of their home institution's facilities, can obtain access to expensive, high-technology tools and the expertise needed to run them (Kaiser, 2001).

HHMI leaders have acknowledged that the kind of research they are proposing for the center is more typically undertaken by biotechnology companies. The Institute will encourage patenting of discoveries made at the center, which may foster the launch of new startup companies. However, the generation of royalty revenues or new private businesses is not a stated goal of the Institute (Kaiser, 2001). Because this project is still in the very early stages of planning, predicting its effectiveness or impact on the broader scientific community is impossible. Nonetheless, it provides a novel and unique model for consideration.

SYNCHROTRON RESOURCES AT THE NATIONAL LABORATORIES

Two institutes from NIH, the NIGMS and the NCI, are providing $23 million over three years to support the design and construction of a user facility at Argonne National Laboratory's Advanced Photon Source (APS), the newest and most advanced synchrotron in the country. After two years of planning, NIGMS and NCI, which represent two-thirds of the life-science synchrotron user community, finalized an agreement early in 2002 to increase synchrotron resources by constructing three new beam lines at Argonne's APS that will be fully operational by 2005. The facility is operated by the University of Chicago, but beam time will be administered by NIH. Half of the beam time will be allocated to peer-reviewed research. NIGMS and NCI grantees will have access to the beam through a peer-review process for research grants. Twenty-five percent of the beam time will be divided between NIGMS and NCI for special projects, and the remaining beam time will be reserved for staff use and maintenance. The NIGMS/NCI facility will be fine-tuned to focus on the aspects of X-rays most useful for biological studies. Demand for beam time is increasing because of such projects as the NIGMS PPSI. NCI is particularly interested in how the synchrotron facilities will advance the study of cancer-related molecules, because an understanding of detailed protein structure will help cancer researchers develop targeted drug therapies. NIGMS and NCI anticipate that information about molecular structures will allow scientists to help develop new medicines and diagnostic techniques. Once construction is complete, operation costs for the beam line are estimated to be $4 million a year, of which NCI has committed $1 million annually. (Cancer Letter, 2001; Softcheck, 2002).

DEFENSE ADVANCED RESEARCH PROJECTS AGENCY

The Defense Advanced Research Projects Agency (DARPA) provides another alternative strategy for undertaking large-scale research projects. DARPA is the central research and development organization for the Department of Defense. It manages and directs selected basic and applied research and development projects for the department, with a focus on projects in which the risk and potential payoff are both very high, and in which success could provide dramatic advances for traditional military roles and missions.

The agency was created in 1958 by President Eisenhower following the Soviet Union's surprise launch of Sputnik (Malakoff, 1999). An investigation blamed delays in the U.S. military satellite program on bureaucratic infighting and an unwillingness to take risks. Intent on keeping the United States at the forefront of technological innovations, Eisenhower ordered Pentagon planners to create an agency that would be completely different from the conventional military research and development structure and, in fact, would serve as a deliberate counterpoint to traditional thinking and approaches. The new agency relied on a small group of experts to look beyond near-term military needs and to fund areas offering great potential to revolutionize military capabilities. Today, the emphasis is still on seeking out and pursuing novel ideas. A list of the agency's founding principles, which are still followed, is provided in Box 3-3.

Best known for its role in developing the Internet (Norberg and O'Neill, 1996), DARPA has funded work focused primarily on computer

BOX 3-3   Founding Principles of DARPA

- Small and flexible establishment
- Flat organization
- Substantial autonomy and freedom from bureaucratic impediments
- Technical staff drawn from world-class scientists and engineers with representation from industry, universities, government laboratories, and federally funded research and development centers.
- Technical staff assigned for 3–5 years and rotated to ensure fresh thinking and perspectives.
- Project based: all efforts are typically 3–5 years long, with a strong focus on end goals. Major technological challenges may be addressed over much longer times, but only as a series of focused steps. Projects are not renewed.
- Necessary supporting personnel (technical, contracting, administrative) are hired on a temporary basis to provide complete flexibility to undertake and abandon an area without problems of sustaining staff. Program managers (the heart of DARPA) are selected to be technically outstanding and entrepreneurial. The best DARPA program managers have always been free-thinking zealots in pursuit of their goals.
- Management is focused on good stewardship of taxpayer funds but imposes little else in terms of rules. Management's job is to enable the program managers.
- A complete acceptance of failure if the payoff for success would have been high enough.

SOURCE: <http://www.darpa.mil>.

and software development, engineering, materials science, microelectronics, and robotics. The agency has had only a limited and very recent interest in basic molecular biology, and most of its biology research relates to just one function—protecting personnel against biological weapons. However, some of this work could potentially have broader implications for biological research, such as novel approaches for DNA sequencing (Alper, 1999) or sophisticated biosensors. Funding for research on this topic began in 1997, with contracts totaling about $50 million going to biotechnology ventures and nonprofit organizations. Although a panel of expert advisors provided some input in launching this program, it is run essentially the same as all other DARPA programs—with hands-on oversight by carefully selected program managers (Marshall, 1997).

With an annual budget of $2 billion, DARPA's small group of about 125 program managers have extensive power to direct high-risk projects that would not normally fare well in peer review. A DARPA program manager will typically spend as much as $40 million on contracts to industry, academic, and government laboratories for one or more projects.

The contracts call for defined deliverables and allow less-promising work to be canceled easily. The agency aims to complete 20 percent of ongoing projects each year, and renewals are not made, although projects are occasionally reformulated for a subsequent attempt. The funded researchers often attend team meetings, file frequent reports, and work cooperatively with other contractors.

Program managers are selected on the basis of their technical expertise and their aspiration to leave their mark on a field. They stay for an average of 4 years and often return to their primary field of research when their term is over. In addition to their technical expertise, they must demonstrate bureaucratic skills, as they must lobby for their portion of the DARPA budget, and be able to move established research communities in a particular direction or create new collaborations in disparate fields. Program managers identify opportunities in science or technology that appear promising, and then make decisions about whom to fund in pursuing the ideas. They may make the latter decisions by probing the network of experts in a field to identify the most appropriate researchers, or by using written specifications to invite experts in the field to apply for funds. Program managers have only two layers of supervision—an office director and the DARPA director, who reports to the Secretary of Defense. These supervisors monitor the performance of the managers and hold them accountable for advancing their fields, but a major criterion for success is positive peer assessment of the manager's performance.

This arrangement is in stark contrast to the current model at NIH, in which peer review is used to select proposals from a competitive pool of grant applications, rather than to assess the performance of program managers. NIH grant management staff generally have a comparatively passive role in project selection. It can also be difficult to determine whether the selected grant portfolios are actually meeting the goals of NIH programs.

Ultimately, the strength of DARPA has been in pursuing innovative research directions to create new fields, or in solving specific technical problems by fostering the development of new technologies. The agency is not responsible for sustaining fields in the long run, as is NIH. Thus, adopting a DARPA model of funding for all NIH programs would be unworkable. However, the addition of some DARPA-like programs to the traditional NIH portfolio might add valuable research that would not otherwise be undertaken.

Indeed, some leaders at NIH, including former director Harold Varmus, have recently expressed interest in adopting some DARPA-like programs at NIH to spark innovation (Malakoff, 1999). Under the leadership of NCI director Richard Klausner, NCI has even launched a pilot program modeled in part after DARPA, as well as other agencies, such as NASA.

The Unconventional Innovations Program (discussed earlier) emulates the DARPA approach by assembling interdisciplinary research teams and pressing them to share information, with the goal of producing breakthroughs in cancer detection technologies. NCI's traditional peer review panels still play a major role in selecting projects, but agency managers are more involved in program oversight than is usual. The program seeks input from and collaboration with investigators that have not traditionally been engaged in biomedical research.

Despite these new developments and the past successes of DARPA, however, such programs do not come without difficult challenges and criticism. One of the greatest challenges to undertaking DARPA-like programs may be the difficulty of recruiting effective managers. The DARPA model works best when the manager is an intellectual peer of the scientists being funded. But for biomedical scientists, a 4-year absence from the laboratory and the resultant lack of published scientific papers during that period could very well be disastrous from a long-range career perspective. In addition, university-based scientists in particular often feel uncomfortable with aggressive supervision and team-dominated research, and biomedical scientists have opposed most initiatives that involve strong external control in the past. Furthermore, it is not uncommon for DARPA-funded projects to fail in meeting their intended goals. This is to be expected, given the high-risk nature of the work, but it may not be a popular approach in other fields. And even when its projects have been successful, DARPA has had difficulty in moving some findings into the military venue or the marketplace (Malakoff, 1999). All of these issues need to be weighed carefully in attempting to emulate the DARPA program in other fields of research.

SUMMARY

As is clear from the examples described in this chapter, the characteristics of large-scale biomedical research projects can vary greatly, even when such research is defined relatively narrowly. However, the examples presented here share many common themes, characteristics, and issues. For example, most are dependent on technology in the sense that they require the use of expensive technologies, the development of novel technologies, refinements to current technologies, or standardization of the way technologies are used and how the information generated is interpreted and analyzed.

Another common feature of the examples described here is a great need for planning, organizational structure, and oversight. The capacity of a large-scale project to efficiently and effectively produce data and other end products that are novel and valuable to the scientific community can be determined by its design and the skill of the individuals who oversee the work. Many of the large-scale projects described here are also quite collaborative and interdisciplinary in nature. For example, the needs for data assessment and technology development mandate the collaboration of scientists who may not have been involved traditionally in biological research, such as engineers, physicists, and computer scientists. This new approach to biology creates additional challenges in communication across disciplines, and can also lead to difficult questions regarding training and career advancement. If interdisciplinary scientists do not fit well into the traditional models of academic science departments, it may be difficult to assess their contribution and compensate them fairly with promotions and tenure. These issues are also relevant to managers of large-scale projects, who are crucial to the success of the effort, but often do not find themselves on traditional academic career paths, and may be given relatively little credit for the accomplishments of the project. These topics are covered in more detail in Chapters 4 through 6.

One issue common to all large-scale biomedical research projects that generate research tools or databases of information is that of accessibility. Concerns are often raised regarding intellectual property rights, open communication among researchers, and public dissemination of data and information. Such concerns may be especially pertinent when for-profit entities are involved in the undertaking. Most projects to date have adopted a policy of making data publicly available, at least in raw form. Research tools and reagents generated through large-scale projects funded by NIH are also often made available to other scientists at cost, but doing so requires a considerable commitment of NIH resources and infrastructure support. Clearly such matters need to be thoroughly addressed before a large-scale project is launched. Chapter 7 examines these issues in greater detail.

The issue of peer review also appears to be extremely important for large-scale projects in biology. Many of the early attempts by NCI to undertake large-scale, directed projects resulted in harsh criticism because of a lack of peer review, which has been fairly standard for NIH funding. Traditionally, NIH decisions about which projects and investigators to fund have been made following peer review of project proposals in grant applications. But peer review could also take other forms, such as reviewing the progress and achievement of grant recipients to determine whether funding should continue or whether the project's goals or objectives should be altered. Peer review might also focus on the performance of program managers who make decisions about which projects and people to fund, as is done under DARPA. Recently, NIH has developed some new large-scale programs that incorporate novel approaches to peer review, whereby steering and advisory committees whose members include scientists not directly involved with the project assess progress and provide advice on future directions. It is still too early to determine how effective these mechanisms are, but thus far they appear to be acceptable to the scientific community. These topics are addressed in more detail in Chapter 4.

4

Funding for Large-Scale Science

Obtaining funding is an essential step in launching any scientific research project. For large-scale projects, the challenges encountered in securing funding to pursue an idea are amplified and in many ways unique. Potential sources of funding include government agencies, philanthropies and other nonprofit organizations, and industry, each of which has its advantages and limitations. In the United States, the federal government has traditionally been the primary funder of large-scale projects, as defined in this report, because of the high costs of such activities.

Not surprisingly, however, the provision of federal funds for large-scale projects has frequently been controversial, both across and within scientific disciplines. The angst across disciplines stems from the sense that large-scale projects funnel an inequitable or unjustified portion of the funds available for science and technology in general to one particular field, thus shortchanging other fields and impeding progress toward useful advances. For example, this argument has been used in debates regarding the proposal to build a superconducting super collider, which was eventually rejected, as well as the proposal for the international space station, which was narrowly passed. The tension within a field stems largely from disagreements over whether large projects or more traditional small-scale projects are the most efficient, economical, and beneficial for moving a field forward in the long run. These questions were widely debated in regard to the Human Genome Project (HGP).

Although the completion of the reference draft of the human genome sequence has been widely hailed as a major achievement that will greatly advance the fields of biology and biomedical research, questions are still being raised as to what role, if any, large-scale projects should have in future biological research. Many believe that smaller conventional, hypothesis-driven projects initiated by individual investigators are the most effective way to advance the field. But given the success of the HGP, there is also great interest in launching similar projects aimed at producing databases and other research tools that could facilitate the progress and potential of smaller, independent projects. Indeed, as noted in Chapter 3, a number of such projects have already been initiated. Thus, perhaps the most relevant question now is not whether the federal government should fund large-scale biology projects, but what the appropriate balance is between funding for large- and small-scale science in biomedical research and how funding for large-scale projects should be allocated. Yet little effort has been made to reach a consensus on the latter question, either in the broad fields of biology and biomedical research or in the more focused field of cancer research.

Even if providing funds for large-scale science is now culturally acceptable in biomedical research, questions remain as to whether NIH is structured to fund such research. There is no agreed-upon method for allocating funds to large-scale projects, and there are many obstacles to overcome in designating funding for such projects, in part because the procedures and mechanisms used to disburse funds are still based on the more traditional approach to science. For example, the current, conventional NIH peer review process for vetting most research proposals is not very favorable to large-scale projects, which may not be hypothesis driven and often have nontraditional goals. But such a vetting process is essential for achieving credibility and buy-in by the scientific community. Knowledgeable members of the community must be able to evaluate adequately and fairly the importance of the large-scale research goals, the feasibility of the plan, the value of the end products, and the level of opportunity to move the field forward. Such evaluation is challenging within the confines of the current system in part because the nature, and thus the assessment, of the goals and deliverables of large-scale biomedical projects are quite different than from those for the customary smaller projects. The organization and planning requirements for large-scale projects are also more elaborate, and therefore likely to require additional oversight and interim endpoints to achieve long-term accountability. Meeting these requirements necessitates additional resources and efforts on the part of the funder as well as the investigator.

This chapter provides an overview of the funding sources and mechanisms available for scientific research, both in general and specifically for biomedical research, with special emphasis on issues that are most relevant to large-scale projects in biomedical research. The discussion begins with a brief review of the history of and process for allocation of federal funds for scientific research. A detailed description of funding for NIH is then presented, followed by a discussion of nonfederal funding of large-scale biomedical research projects. Issues associated with international collaborations are also examined.

HISTORY OF FEDERAL SUPPORT FOR SCIENTIFIC RESEARCH

The U.S government has often used its monetary resources to pursue matters of national interest. As the country's foundations were being laid, scientific research was not a national priority because the nation relied less on matters of science than it does today. But although federal scientific pursuits had a slow start, strong foundations were formed in the early nineteenth century that made possible the significant momentum in government sponsorship of public-based scientific endeavors experienced in the early part of the twentieth century (see Appendix). While early government investment in scientific research programs focused on agriculture, national security, exploration, and commerce, many private foundations, such as Carnegie, Rockefeller, and Smithsonian, were supporting a variety of university-based basic research projects. That dichotomy is no longer true, as the U.S. federal government now supports the majority of basic scientific research undertaken at the nation's universities.

The earliest federal support for civilian research was authorized in the 1800s, and included large-scale projects such as the U.S. Coast Survey and the U.S. Geological Survey. However, these initial efforts did not support the scientific education, training, and basic research that is now the hallmark of universities. The first federal support for basic research within universities was initiated by the creation of the Department of Agriculture and the Land Grant Colleges. A series of congressional acts, starting with the Morrill Act of 1862, provided the mechanism by which scientists at universities could propose research projects and obtain federal funding to carry them out. These developments played a substantial role in the formation of a number of biological sciences in the United States, including bacteriology, biochemistry, and genetics (Goldberg, 1995). The creation of NIH eventually led to an analogous impact on biomedical research when it began providing federal funds for extramural projects at universities. Similarly, the creation of NCI in 1937 was instrumental in launching a federally sponsored campaign to understand and eliminate human cancer.

The period of time surrounding World War II had a particularly significant impact on the government's investment in university-based scientific research and its willingness to underwrite big-science projects. During the decade from 1940 to 1950, several key events facilitated the creation or expansion of science-oriented agencies, such as the Office of

Naval Research, the National Science Foundation (NSF), and NIH, whose main objectives became the sponsorship of public research. A key initial impetus for the expansion of federally sponsored scientific research was Vannevar Bush's 1945 report to the President—*Science: The Endless Frontier*—but other leaders also played important roles in developing the current mechanisms for federal support of science, particularly with respect to the more applied fields of research.[1] (For a detailed review, see Appendix.) The resultant changes ensured that federal funding for university-based scientific research would become the accepted and expected norm that it is today. These changes also paved the way for federal support of future big-science projects in such fields as high-energy physics, space science, and biology.

ALLOCATION OF FEDERAL FUNDS FOR SCIENTIFIC RESEARCH

The process for appropriating federal funds is both complex and treacherous. The separation of powers between the executive and legislative branches of the U.S. government makes it difficult to ascribe responsibility for any particular government action. Decisions regarding budgets and funding priorities are made through complex procedures that are influenced by many factors and federal entities. Determining funding priorities in a fluctuating social and economic environment is difficult, and by its very nature controversial. The U.S. government must determine how much money should be allocated for scientific research as a whole, and how to divide that money among the various claimants in the science and technology community (Green, 1995). Yet broad priority setting is generally resisted by the recipients of federal funding because it orders the importance of research investments in ways that groups within the scientific community often do not support (Office of Technology Assessment, 1991; McGeary and Merrill, 1999). The process is inherently contentious because priority setting creates winners and losers. Although American science is unparalleled in its scale and scope compared with that of other nations, the publicly financed sector exists in an economy of scarcity because scientists and institutions will always have more ideas for research projects than can be funded (Greenberg, 2001). In resisting priority setting, the scientific community aims to maintain high levels of funding for all fields, instead of risking cuts in any particular one.

There are few established methods for comparing, evaluating, and ranking research programs regardless of their size, although criteria have been proposed (Office of Technology Assessment, 1991; see Box 4-1). Even

---

[1] Vannevar Bush made a strong distinction between basic and applied research, and generally did not advocate government support of applied research.

BOX 4-1   A Statement from the Scientific Community on the Evaluation of Competing Scientific Initiatives

The following criteria were proposed in 1988 for evaluating competing scientific initiatives. They are presented here (in abridged form) in the three categories developed by the authors.

Scientific Merit

1. Scientific objective and significance
   Example: What are the key scientific issues addressed by the initiative?
2. Breadth of interest
   Examples: Why is the initiative important or critical to the discipline proposing it? What impact will the science involved have on other disciplines?
3. Potential for new discoveries and understanding
   Examples: Will the initiative provide powerful new techniques for probing nature? What advances beyond previous measurements can be expected with respect to accuracy, sensitivity, comprehensiveness, and range? In what ways will the initiative advance the understanding of widely occurring natural processes and stimulate modeling and theoretical description of these processes?
4. Uniqueness
   Example: What are the special reasons for proposing this initiative? Could the desired knowledge be obtained in other ways? Is a special time schedule necessary for performing the initiative?

Social Benefits

1. Contribution to scientific awareness or improvement of the human condition
   Examples: Are the goals of the initiative related to broader public objectives such as human welfare, economic growth, or national security? Will the results assist in planning for the future? What is the potential for stimulating technological developments that have application beyond this particular initiative? Will the initiative contribute to public understanding of the goals and accomplishments of science?
2. Contribution to international understanding
   Example: Will the initiative contribute to international collaboration and understanding?
3. Contribution to national pride and prestige
   Example: Will the initiative create public pride because of the magnitude of the challenge, the excitement of the endeavor, or the nature of the results?

Programmatic Concerns

1. Feasibility and readiness
   Examples: Is the initiative technologically feasible? Are there adequate plans and facilities to receive, process, analyze, store, distribute, and use data at the expected rate of acquisition?
2. Scientific logistics and infrastructure
   Examples: What are the long-term requirements for special facilities or field op-

BOX 4-1 *continued*

erations? What current and long-term infrastructure is required to support the initiative and the processing and analysis of data?

3. Community commitment and readiness
   Example: In what ways will the scientific community participate in the operation of the initiative and the analysis of the results?

4. Institutional implications
   Examples: In what ways will the initiative stimulate research and education? What opportunities and challenges will the initiative present for universities, federal laboratories, and industrial contractors? What will be the impact of the initiative on federally sponsored science? Can some current activities be curtailed if the initiative is successful?

5. International involvement
   Example: Are there commitments for programmatic support from other nations or international organizations?

6. Cost of the proposed initiative
   Examples: What are the total costs, by year, to the Federal budget? What portion of the total costs will be borne by other nations?

SOURCE: Office of Technology Assessment, 1991. Adapted from: John A. Dutton and Lawson Crewe, 1988.

within a discipline, distribution of funds can be contentious, as demonstrated by the 1995 National Research Council (NRC) study that produced the report *Setting Priorities in Space Research: An Experiment in Methodology*, in which no consensus was reached on how to make allocations. The challenges associated with allocating funds across scientific fields are even greater. No single organization looks across the federal research system to determine priorities, and there is currently no formal or explicit mechanism for evaluating the total research portfolio of the federal government in terms of progress toward national objectives. Mechanisms that may help determine priorities include the individual agency advisory committees (see Box 4-2) and peer review procedures, the Office of Science and Technology Policy and other White House advisory committees, and the NRC system. Even with these mechanisms in place, however, there is no way to avoid competition among the various claims on federal science funds or to balance the federal research portfolio systematically.

As described in more detail below, a variety of unrelated agency budgets could be in competition for the funds available under the jurisdiction of an individual appropriations committee, and no single subcommittee is responsible for all science funding agencies, making it very

---

BOX 4-2   Federal Advisory Committees at the National Institutes of Health

NIH maintains more than 140 chartered advisory committees (the largest number of federal advisory committees of any Executive Branch agency), authorized by the Public Health Service Act. This Act authorizes scientific and technical peer review of biomedical and behavioral research grant and cooperative agreement applications, research and development contracts, and research conducted at NIH through advisory committees. Federal advisory committees follow the Federal Advisory Committee Act (FACA). The advisory committees used by NIH fall into four categories:

• Initial/integrated review groups (IRGs) and special emphasis panels (SEPs)—Provide scientific and technical merit review, which is the first level of peer review of research grant applications and contract proposals.
• National advisory councils and boards (NACs)—Perform the second level of peer review for research grant applications, and offer advice and recommendations on policy and program development, program implementation, evaluation, and other matters of significance to the mission and goals of the respective Institutes or Centers. Provide oversight of research conducted by each Institute's or Center's intramural program.
• Boards of scientific counselors (BSCs)—Review and evaluate the research programs and investigators of the intramural laboratories.
• Program advisory committees (PACs)—Provide advice on specific research programs and future research needs and opportunities, and identify and evaluate extramural initiatives.

SOURCE: <http://www1.od.nih.gov/cmo/CmoOv.html>.

---

difficult to prioritize across disciplines. The NRC (1995) identified this predicament as a major obstacle in allocating federal funds for science and technology equitably and appropriately across the various fields and agencies. The report recommended changes to the process that would allow presentation and examination of the entire, comprehensive science and technology budget before it is disaggregated among the various committees and subcommittees. Only recently have Congress and the Administration begun to discuss the balance of funding among fields. For the fiscal year (FY) 2001 budget cycle, the Bush Administration stated for the first time that balance would be an explicit criterion in developing its budget request. The budget contained a component called "Federal Science and Technology," which was meant to represent investment in new knowledge and know-how. This was a break from tradition, but still does not enable priority setting among fields (National Research Council, 2001a). Thus, the NRC report recommended that the executive branch and Congress institutionalize processes for conducting and acting on an integrated analysis of the federal budget for research, by field as well as by agency, national purpose, and other perspectives.

One ongoing change in budget allocations is the effort by the Office of Management and Budget (OMB) to apply stricter performance measures in funding federal research agencies based on the Government Performance and Results Act (GPRA) of 1993 (Hafner, 2002). GPRA requires agencies to manage and budget according to performance standards as a way of promoting efficiency, accountability, and effectiveness in government spending. However, it is still unclear to what extent Congress will adopt more definitive guidelines, with an emphasis on output, for scientific research. In the past, Congress has been amenable to investing in undifferentiated science, with knowledge as the outcome. Indeed, GRPA has caused consternation among the research agencies because few have had any experience in actually measuring the results of their programs, and they are unaccustomed to the increased scrutiny. Many researchers have argued that the results of ongoing basic research cannot be benchmarked or measured (Lekowski, 1999).

A 1999 report addressing the issue of assessing research in compliance with GPRA agreed that basic research cannot be measured directly on an annual basis because its outcomes are unpredictable, and there is generally a significant time delay between the generation of new knowledge and its practical application (National Research Council, 1999). However, the report did suggest that measures of quality, relevance, and leadership are sound indicators of eventual usefulness and can be reported regularly while research is in progress. The report also encouraged benchmarking of programs in one agency against other federal programs, as well as international benchmarking, as a measure for fostering quality and leadership in a given field of research. The report made two additional major recommendations: that research programs also be graded on whether they perform an effective education and training function, and that interagency programs be graded according to how well they are coordinated.

The FY 2003 federal budget marks the first year that OMB has actually linked management performance with research budget priorities (Softcheck, 2002). The process for using the new performance criteria and standards for applied research and development (R&D) was piloted with the Department of Energy (DOE) (Hafner, 2002). Standards for evaluating basic R&D are still in development, with plans to implement them in FY 2004 across all federal research agencies. Assessment parameters will be refined in consultation with a variety of scientific bodies, such as the National Academies' Committee on Science, Engineering, and Public Policy (COSEPUP).

As part of the new focus on performance, OMB recently released a red/yellow/green scorecard for each federal agency (with red being the lowest score). Almost 80 percent of those reviewed received red scores in the five rating categories. Only one agency, NSF, received a green score in one of the five categories—for financial management (Softcheck, 2002). However, a recent follow-up study by COSEPUP also examined the ways in which federal agencies that support science and engineering research are responding to GPRA (National Academies, 2001). The committee found that although there is significant variation in responses, NIH, NSF, the Department of Defense (DOD), DOE, and the National Aeronautics and Space Administration (NASA) have all taken steps to develop reporting procedures to comply with GPRA requirements. The committee also concluded that some agencies were using GPRA to improve their operations, but that oversight bodies needed clearer procedures to validate and verify the agency evaluations, and that communication between oversight bodies and the agencies was not adequate.

An overview of the process for appropriating and allocating federal funds in the United States is shown in Figure 4-1. Briefly, the President, in conjunction with OMB, submits a detailed budget that includes many line-item requests about 15 months prior to the start of the budget's fiscal year. OMB crafts the budgets of research programs to reflect the priorities of the President, and attempts to compare the projected costs, benefits, and risks of certain programs to set realistic targets for the budget. The President's budget is submitted to both the House and Senate budget committees. These two committees review the budget and make changes to broad funding areas, called functions, in the areas of health, defense, civilian R&D, and so on. Congressional authorizing committees[2] then can either authorize or not authorize (as nearly occurred with the space station) the use of the funds by specific government agencies and programs. The revised budget is next given to the House and Senate full appropriations committees and is divided among the 13 corresponding appropriation subcommittees,[3] which are mirrored on the House and Senate sides (see Table 4-1). Although specific budget items may have been outlined by the President, the budget committees, the authorizing committees, and the appropriations committees have the decisive influence over the funds distributed to R&D agencies.

Each of the 13 appropriations subcommittees from the House and Senate writes a bill that is submitted back to the respective full committee, and the bills are taken to the House or Senate floor. Once the bills have

---

[2] Authorizing committees supervise the activities of agencies under their jurisdiction and pass laws (authorization bills) directing those activities and setting nonbinding ceilings for their budgets.

[3] The appropriations committees set the actual budgets of all agencies in the government.

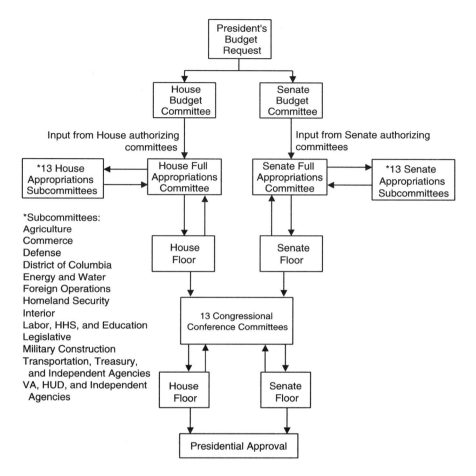

FIGURE 4-1   Federal budget approval process.

been approved, they go to a congressional conference committee made up of House and Senate members from the corresponding appropriations subcommittees. The further revised individual bills, often a compromise between House and Senate versions, are taken back to the floor and submitted for a vote. If approved, each bill goes back to the President for signing. As the President signs the final bills, they become laws. The "budget" for R&D is contained in the aggregate of appropriations bills passed for the year.

One limitation of this system that may be especially relevant to the funding of large-scale research projects is that federal appropriations are

TABLE 4-1   Selected Congressional Appropriations Committee
Jurisdictions

| Appropriations Committee or Subcommittee Name | Committee Jurisdiction | |
	Senate	House
Agriculture	1. **Department of Agriculture** (except Forest Service) 2. Farm Credit Administration 3. Commodity Futures Trading Commission 4. Food and Drug Administration (DHHS)	1. Adulteration of seeds, insect pests, and protection of birds and animals in forest reserves 2. Agriculture generally 3. **Agricultural and industrial chemistry** 4. **Agricultural colleges and experiment stations** 5. Agricultural economics and research 6. Agricultural education extension services 7. Agricultural production and marketing and stabilization of prices of agricultural products and commodities (not including distribution outside the United States) 8. Animal industry and diseases of animals 9. Crop insurance and soil conservation 10. Dairy industry 11. Entomology and plant quarantine 12. Extension of farm credit and farm security 13. Forestry in general, and forest reserves other than those created from the public domain 14. Human nutrition and home economics 15. Inspection of livestock and meat products 16. Plant industry, soils, and agricultural engineering 17. Rural electrification 18. Commodities exchanges 19. Rural development

TABLE 4-1 *continued*

Defense	1. **Department of Defense—** Military: Departments of Army, Navy (including Marine Corps), Air Force, and Office of Secretary of Defense (except Military Construction) 2. The Central Intelligence Agency 3. Intelligence Community Oversight	1. **Department of Defense—** Military: Departments of Army, Navy (including Marine Corps), Air Force 2. **Office of Secretary of Defense, and Defense Agencies** (except military construction) 3. Central Intelligence Agency 4. Intelligence Community Staff
Energy and Water Development	1. **Department of Energy** (except Economic Regulatory Administration; Energy Information Administration; Strategic Petroleum Reserve; Naval Petroleum and Oil Shale Reserves; Emergency Preparedness, Office of Hearings and Appeals; Fossil Energy Research and Development; Energy Conservation; Alternative Fuels Production and Related Matters) 2. **Department of Defense—Civil; Department of the Army, Corps of Engineers—Civil** 3. Department of the Interior, Bureau of Reclamation, Related Agencies 4. Appalachian Regional Commission 5. Appalachian Regional Development Programs 6. Delaware River Basin Commission 7. Interstate Commission on the Potomac River Basin 8. National Council on Public Works Improvement 9. Nuclear Regulatory Commission 10. Office of Water Policy 11. Susquehanna River Basin Commission 12. Tennessee Valley Authority	1. **Department of Energy** (except the Economic Regulatory Administration; Energy Information Administration, Office of Hearings and Appeals, Strategic Petroleum Reserve, Naval Petroleum and Oil Shale Reserves, Fossil Energy Research and Development, Clean Coal Technology, Energy Conservation, Alternative Fuels Production and Related Matters) 2. **Department of Defense— Civil** 3. **Department of the Army, Corps of Engineers—Civil** 4. Department of the Interior, Bureau of Reclamation 5. Central Utah Project, Related Agencies 6. Appalachian Regional Commission 7. Defense Nuclear Facilities Safety Board 8. Nuclear Regulatory Commission 9. Nuclear Waste Technical Review Board 10. Tennessee Valley Authority
Labor, Health and Human Services, and Education	1. Department of Education (except Indian Education Activities) 2. **Department of Health and**	1. Department of Education 2. **Department of Health and Human Services** (except Food and Drug

(continued on next page)

TABLE 4-1 *continued*

	Human Services (except Food and Drug Administration, Indian Education Activities, Indian Health Services and Facilities, Office of Consumer Affairs) 3. Department of Labor, Related Agencies 4. Corporation for Public Broadcasting 5. Federal Mediation and Conciliation Service 6. Federal Mine Safety and Health Review Commission 7. National Commission on Libraries and Information Science 8. National Council on the Handicapped 9. National Labor Relations Board 10. National Mediation Board 11. Occupational Safety and Health Review Commission 12. Medicare Payment Advisory Commission 13. Railroad Retirement Board 14. Soldiers' and Airmen's Home 15. U.S. Institute of Peace	Administration, Indian Health Services and Facilities, Office of Consumer Affairs) 3. Department of Labor, Related Agencies 4. Armed Forces Retirement Home 5. Corporation for National and Community Service (VISTA and seniors programs only) 6. Corporation for Public Broadcasting 7. Federal Mediation and Conciliation Service 8. Federal Mine Safety and Health Review Commission 9. National Commission on Libraries and Information Science 10. National Council on Disability 11. National Education Goals Panel 12. National Foundation on the Arts and Humanities (Office of Library Services) 13. National Labor Relations Board 14. National Mediation Board 15. Occupational Safety and Health Review Commission 16. Medicare Payment Advisory Commission 17. Railroad Retirement Board 18. Social Security Administration 19. U.S. Institute of Peace
Veterans Affairs, Housing and Urban Development, Independent Agencies	1. Department of Veterans Affairs 2. Department of Housing and Urban Development 3. American Battle Monuments Commission 4. Cemeterial Expenses, Army (Department of Defense) 5. Consumer Information Center (General Services Administration)	1. Department of Veterans Affairs 2. Department of Housing and Urban Development, Independent Agencies 3. American Battle Monuments Commission 4. Cemeterial Expenses, Army (Department of Defense) 5. Community Development

TABLE 4-1 *continued*

6. Consumer Product Safety Commission	Financial Institutions (Treasury)
7. Council on Environmental Quality and Office of Environmental Quality	6. Consumer Information Center (General Services Administration)
8. Department of the Treasury, Office of Revenue Sharing	7. Consumer Product Safety Commission
9. Environmental Protection Agency	8. Corporation for National and Community Service
10. Federal Emergency Management Agency	9. Council on Environmental Quality and Office of Environmental Quality
11. Federal Home Loan Bank Board	10. Court of Veterans Appeals
12. **National Aeronautics and Space Administration**	11. Environmental Protection Agency
13. National Commission on Air Quality	12. Federal Emergency Management Agency
14. National Credit Union Administration	13. **National Aeronautics and Space Administration**
15. National Institute of Building Sciences	14. National Credit Union Administration
16. **National Science Foundation**	15. **National Science Foundation**
17. Neighborhood Reinvestment Corporation	16. Neighborhood Reinvestment Corporation
18. Office of Consumer Affairs (Health and Human Services)	17. Office of Consumer Affairs (Health and Human Services)
19. Office of Science and Technology Policy	18. Office of Science and Technology Policy
20. Selective Service System	19. Resolution Trust Corporation: Office of Inspector General
	20. Selective Service System

NOTE: Agencies in boldface are ones that commonly fund science research activities. Agencies within a committee's jurisdiction may compete for the budgetary funds authorized to their appropriations committee.
SOURCE: Congressional Yellow Book (2001).

made on an annual basis. In contrast, most research projects last for several years, and large-scale projects in particular may require long-term planning. During lean budget years, big-ticket items may be appealing targets for cuts, and thus the funding for large-scale projects may be especially vulnerable to funding instability. DOD does have some multiyear budgets, but this is a rare exception. Most science agencies, such as NIH, must make difficult decisions about how to disburse funds among new projects and those already in progress. As a result, when budgets are lower than expected, scientists may have to make do with fewer resources than they had anticipated on the basis of funding commitments in previous years, and some new initiatives may also be eliminated.

NIH may be especially vulnerable to these fluctuations because of its allocation process and "commitment base." NSF and several of the defense agencies generally sequester some funds at the time of award, but NIH has not chosen this approach. This policy can lead to problems if budget growth rates are lower than anticipated. This was a main cause of difficulties experienced in 1990–1993, when a rapid rise in cost per grant took place concurrently with an administrative decision to lengthen grants to reduce instability for investigators. NIH has also occasionally undertaken standardized "downward negotiations" for ongoing projects, which are actually unilateral after-the-fact budget cuts in ongoing grants to free funds for new grants. From time to time, OMB has urged NIH to adopt a "pay as you go" process. This would not eliminate the problem, but would make it less acute and render funding somewhat more predictable. NIH's policy may be appropriate given its almost monotonic budget growth history, but when its budget hits steady state or declines, NIH has more difficult decisions to make than other agencies.

Another important vulnerability for federally funded large-scale research projects is that they may be "on–off" items that often require rapid increases in specific line items and so become quite conspicuous in the budget process, which usually starts from a stable baseline. For example, a large-scale cyclotron project must be fully funded to build and operate the cyclotron, or there is no point in funding the project at all. The rapid rise of specific line items is a serious issue because budget analysts at OMB, throughout the Department of Health and Human Services (DHHS), and on the appropriation subcommittees are trained to look for percent increases that stand out, as these require special justification. However, it could be argued that this difficulty is not as meaningful to many large-scale projects in biology as it is to large projects in other scientific fields. For instance, if the National Human Genome Research Institute had been given only 80 percent of its budget, it could still have generated DNA sequence data, but the Human Genome Project would have taken longer because fewer sequencers and staff would have been available for the project.

NIH FUNDING

The majority of federal funding for biomedical research is allocated through NIH. The processes through which federal dollars are appropriated to NIH and then dispensed to a vast array of research projects through the various Institutes is also quite complex, as briefly summarized in this section. Indeed, a 1998 report of the Institute of Medicine reviews the procedures for priority setting at NIH, and makes recommendations for improving the process (Institute of Medicine, 1998).

NIH has been the recipient of considerable increases in funding in recent years (Varmus, 1999) as a result of strong support for biomedical research in Congress and among the public, based on the assumption that there is a direct relationship between investment and improved treatments for disease[4] (Haley, 2000). Along with this growth in funding have come increased interest and pressure from advocacy groups, as well as Congress, to distribute the funds for research on the basis of relative disease burden in the United States (Davis, 2000; Varmus, 1999), in addition to the traditional criterion of scientific opportunity. While a recent study found that the amount of NIH funding for specific diseases was associated with some measurements of disease burden (Gross et al., 1999), attempting to distribute funds using this parameter is immensely complex, in part because basic research can be quite difficult to categorize according to specific diseases. Large-scale projects that have broad scientific goals and aim to produce databases, new technologies, and other research tools may be especially difficult to categorize in this way.

Large-scale research projects that require unusually large sums of money over several years, are not hypothesis driven, and aim to develop databases and technologies for use in future research present many additional challenges to the traditional funding mechanisms and procedures at NIH. Unless NIH develops a specific initiative to solicit large-scale projects for a particular field of research, investigators are likely to find it very difficult to overcome obstacles associated with peer review and restrictions on award sizes in the current system. Many established scientists, in speaking before the National Cancer Policy Board, have borne witness to these difficulties encountered in their own recent attempts to obtain NIH funding for large-scale projects (see Box 4-3). These issues are elaborated in greater detail in the following sections, which provide an overview of the steps involved in NIH appropriations and disbursements.

Congressional Appropriations to NIH

NIH is made up of 24 Institutes and Centers, each with a separate, annual budget from Congress. Each Institute within NIH determines how it will allocate its designated resources and funds, but the NIH director plays an active role in shaping the overall budget, activities, and outlook

---

[4] This correlation is questionable, and several recent studies suggest that behavioral changes and social awareness can have a greater impact on the population's health than the discovery of new treatments (Funding First Collection, 2000).

BOX 4-3   Case Examples of Challenges in Funding and Launching Large-Scale Research Projects in Biology

CASE #1: Functional Proteomics

Dr. Edward Harlow, dean for research and chair of the Department of Biological Chemistry and Pharmacology at Harvard Medical School, spoke about his experiences at a quarterly meeting of the National Cancer Policy Board in January 2001. His goal is to produce a functional copy of a proteome by identifying all full-length open reading frames and putting them in a vector system through which any gene or genes of interest could be expressed at will. Recent advances in technology, including automation methodologies and new cloning strategies that can be used on a genome-wide scale, have made such an undertaking potentially feasible. Harvard Medical School and grants from NIH have funded the initial pilot stage of the work for about 3 years. Dr. Harlow reported that preliminary results in a series of different organisms are very encouraging; thus, he believes that the methodology, once verified for accuracy, could be used for any conceivable laboratory screen, including protein binding screens and drug candidate screens. Thus far, the project has expended about $6 million, and the proof-of-principle and pilot stage of the work has now been completed. Completion of the full-scale project will cost an estimated $50 million.

In his search for funding, Dr. Harlow has presented the idea and preliminary results to officials at NIH, pharmaceutical companies, and foundations in both the United States and Great Britain. Although much interest in the project was expressed, he concluded that there is currently no mechanism for launching a project with this sort of framework through any of the normal funding mechanisms. In particular, he noted that there is no funding opportunity for proof-of-principle experiments, and there is no process in place for vetting potential large-scale projects vying for funding. He pointed out that even the provision of seed money and laboratory space by Harvard Medical School was quite unusual.

To date, Dr. Harlow had not yet obtained funding for the full-scale project. Numerous strategies for funding the project are currently being pursued. The construction of several smaller sets of useful genes has been completed, and they now are in use. The plan is to make the end products of the project widely available to the scientific community without intellectual property restraints.

CASE #2: Functional Genomics of the Brain

Dr. Nathaniel Heintz, Howard Hughes Investigator at Rockefeller University, also addressed the National Cancer Policy Board in January 2001. His project, called GENSAT, is aimed at studying functional genomics in the brain. Brain tissue contains tens of thousands of cell types, each very different in morphology and function, which must be complexly interconnected for the organ to work properly. Knowing the precise constellation of cells that express a particular gene of interest can provide very important information about protein function. Dr. Heintz has developed a novel methodology for obtaining this type of information for any given gene by producing specialized transgenic mice, at a very reduced cost per gene (about $5,000) compared with traditional approaches to creating and studying transgenic mice ($50,000 or more per gene). Using this new methodology, which is based on homologous recombination of marked genes through the manipulation of very large DNA con-

BOX 4-3 *continued*

structs, it is conceivable that thousands of novel genes in the brain can be studied in a relatively short period of time.

The basic research that led to the development of this technology was funded by the Howard Hughes Medical Institute (HHMI). However, HHMI was not the appropriate agency to fund a large-scale project aimed at applying the technology, with an estimated cost of $25 million over 5 years (to study 1,000 genes/year). As a result, Dr. Heintz searched for other potential funding mechanisms. His first idea was to form an academic consortium. He contacted about 25 leading neuroscientists, and found that while many were interested in the project, few volunteered to participate in such a consortium. He also considered approaching industry for funding, but decided against this route because of intellectual property concerns—he wanted the resultant database to be free and open to the public. In addition, he noted past difficulties in turning to companies to accomplish his research goals. "If you lose control and if the science gets off track, it's very hard to get it back on track in a company setting, unless you are the founder. And . . . I didn't want to found a company," he said.

In response to positive feedback from NIH staff regarding the technology, Dr. Heintz decided to present his idea to Jerry Fischbach, then director of the National Institute of Neurological Disorders and Stroke (NINDS). He had heard from colleagues that cooperative agreements were very complex and difficult to administer, so he investigated the contract mechanism, whereby decisions would be made directly within NINDS with considerable influence from the director. There was no preexisting call for contracts in this area, but after about 1 year, he and his colleagues Mary E. Hatten and Alexandra Joyyner were awarded a contract for the project, despite difficulties encountered during the review process as a result of the novelty of the technology.

Although fortunate to receive funding, Dr. Heintz noted many challenges associated with the contract mechanism. For example, every contract has a "go-no go" clause in the first year of the contract. As a result, Dr. Heintz needed to obtain a commitment of new laboratory space and numerous animal facilities on extremely short notice, and was under pressure to hire 15 new staff members very quickly. He pointed out that a lag time of even a few months could be devastating for maintaining the contract funding, in sharp contrast to a more traditional 5-year grant, under which a delay of a few months would not have a major impact on funding stability. Thus, he noted that preliminary funding and other support from the host academic institution and its leadership are critical in trying to initiate a large-scale project within academia.

In addition, a great deal of influence over the decision as to whether to continue contract funding rests in the hands of a single person, the program officer, at NIH. Initially, Dr. Heintz felt confident that he had the support of the NINDS director, but Dr. Fischbach has since left NIH, so if the priorities of the new director are different, his funding could be more vulnerable. He noted that recruiting and retaining quality staff to run the project in the face of funding instability was a serious obstacle. As a result, he concluded, "I think the contract mode has strong advantages towards getting [a large-scale project] funded, but the security of the funding is so tenuous that, having done it, I probably would not go through the contract process again."

(continued on next page)

BOX 4-3 *continued*

CASE #3: Genetics of Breast Cancer

Dr. Barbara Weber, director of the Cancer Genomics Program at the University of Pennsylvania Cancer Center, addressed the National Cancer Policy Board in July 2001. The objective of one of her projects is to identify genes that modify the activity of the BRCA1 gene, and thus affect the penetrance of hereditary mutations in BRCA-1 that lead to breast cancer. Many scientists are searching for such "modifier genes," but most use a candidate gene approach in which genes of known function with some relationship to BRCA1 are tested. Because this approach could miss genes that have yet to be characterized or associated with BRCA1, Dr. Weber favors a whole-genome linkage study to identify candidate modifier genes. This method involves genotyping many markers along each of the chromosomes in several hundred people to look for inheritance patterns that correlate with the occurrence of familial breast cancer. A pilot study in which markers along chromosomes 4 and 5 were analyzed in about 25 women led to the identification of a locus on chromosome 5 that may contain a BRCA1 modifier gene (Nathanson et al., 2002).

Dr. Weber has sought funding for the full-scale, whole-genome project from both NIH and the Sanger Center in the United Kingdom, but has not been successful in securing funding from those sources because of the high-risk nature of the project. She submitted proposals to the genotyping Centers sponsored by NIH, knowing that it would be more efficient to carry out the large-scale genotyping project in a Center that was already set up and staffed for such a purpose, rather than trying to establish new facilities and staff at her own institution. (Resources and facilities for high-throughput genotyping are currently available nationally through the National Heart, Lung, and Blood Institute Mammalian Genotyping Service [MGS] and the Center for Inherited Disease Research [CIDR], which were established as a service for research efforts focused on identifying genetic loci involved in human disease. CIDR is a joint effort by eight participating institutes at NIH, including NCI, with the National Human Genome Research Institute serving as the lead agency and manager of the facility.) Dr. Weber believes that the project could be accomplished for about $400,000 by one of the genotyping Centers on a fee-for-service basis, or by a private company if she could obtain the funding from an NIH Institute or other source. However, the traditional funding mechanisms of NIH do not favor such high-risk, open-ended projects that search for unknown targets.

---

of the agency.[5] The director has primary responsibility for advising the President on the annual White House budget request to Congress, based on extensive discussions with the Institute directors. The formulation and presentation of the NIH budget provide a framework within which priorities are identified, reviewed, and justified. The House and Senate appropriations committees also play a major role in NIH priority setting, often appropriating more than the President's budget requests and putting forth specific funding directives (Institute of Medicine, 1998).

---

[5] "Setting Research Priorities at the National Institutes of Health"; see <http://www.nih.gov/news/ResPriority/priority.htm#Funds>.

The NIH director has two additional tools for identifying and funding NIH research efforts. First, the director may transfer up to 1 percent of the total NIH budget among Institutes, although such a move is likely to be controversial. Second, the director has a discretionary fund. Both tools could potentially be used to launch particularly promising or urgent areas of research. Transfer funding typically follows extensive discussions with the Institute directors, as well as advice from outside experts, to identify particular research initiatives that reflect NIH-wide priorities or an emerging need that requires a timely infusion of funds. DHHS, the Administration, and congressional appropriations subcommittees are then notified of NIH's intent to transfer the money. No single Institute can lose more than 1 percent of its appropriated funds in this process.

The director's discretionary fund is used to support specific research opportunities that arise during the course of a year that would otherwise have to wait until the following year for funding. This fund provides a mechanism for early research support by giving additional funding to one or more Institutes. The NIH director can also use these funds to respond to specific requests from Congress or to a public health emergency.

NCI is in a unique position within NIH as a result of the budgetary bypass provision of the National Cancer Act, which permits NCI to submit annual budget requests directly to the President. The NCI director prepares the bypass budget with input from a variety of advisory boards and committees (see Table 4-2). The NIH director and DHHS secretary may comment on the NCI bypass budget, but they cannot change the proposal. The NCI director also prepares another budget that goes through the usual channels of review at NIH and DHHS before being transmitted to OMB, and this is generally the budget that becomes the basis for appropriations hearings, but the bypass budget is an independent input to OMB and the appropriators. Within NCI, the major budget activities fall into several broad categories, as shown in Box 4-4.

Once the actual amount of congressional appropriations is known, final allocations and funding decisions are made by an executive committee[6] within each Institute. Considerations in determining program allocations include congressional mandates; new scientific opportunities; new

---

[6] The NCI executive committee consists of representatives from the Office of the Director, including the director, the deputy director, the associate director for Management, the associate director for Financial Management, the deputy director for Extramural Science, the director of Division of Extramural Activities, the seven division directors of the Institute, the associate director of the Frederick Cancer Research and Development Center, the co-chairs of the Board of Scientific Counselors, the chair of the Board of Scientific Advisors, the chair of the Intramural Advisory Board, the chair of the Extramural Advisory Board, and an Executive Secretary. All major organizational and operating decisions affecting NCI are made by the executive committee.

TABLE 4-2   NCI Advisory Boards and Groups

Name	Structure
President's Cancer Panel, Established by Congress December 1971[a]	3 members, including 2 distinguished scientists/physicians, appointed by the President to serve 3-year terms.
National Cancer Advisory Board, Established by Congress the National Cancer Act in 1937; restructured by of 1971[a]	18 members, appointed for 6-year terms by the President; includes 12 nonvoting ex officio members representing DHHS, OSTP, NIH, VA, OSHA, Secretary of Labor, FDA, EPA, the Consumer Product Safety Commission, DOD Health Affairs, and DOE.
Board of Scientific Advisors	35 authorities knowledgeable in the fields of laboratory, clinical, and biometric research; clinical cancer treatment; cancer etiology; and cancer prevention and control. Members are appointed by the NCI director for terms of up to 5 years.
Board of Scientific Counselors, Established by NCI director October 1995	60 authorities knowledgeable in the fields of laboratory, clinical, and biometric research; clinical cancer treatment; cancer etiology; and cancer prevention and control. Appointed by the NCI director for 5-year terms.
Advisory Committee to the Director[a]	Members: • NCI director (as chair), NCI deputy director, deputy director for NCI extramural science, director of NCI extramural activities • NCAB, BSC chair(s) and co-chair(s), BSA chair(s) and co-chair(s) • Consumer representative, NCI director's Consumer Liaison Group chair

Function	Meetings
Monitors the development and execution of the activities of the National Cancer Program, and reports directly to the President.	Quarterly

- Advises, assists, consults with, and makes recommendations to the Secretary of DHHS, the NIH director, and the NCI director with respect to the activities carried out by NCI, including reviewing and recommending for support grants and cooperative agreements, following technical and scientific peer review. Provides the second tier of peer review for grants funded by NCI.
- The Special Actions subcommittee reviews any grant with an extraordinary situation, as indicated by an NCI staff member, that requires Board advice, approval, or clarification. These situations include grant review disagreements between a program director and an integrated review group (IRG), and grants that involve biohazard, animal welfare, or human subject concerns.

Quarterly

- Advises the NCI director, deputy director for extramural science, and NCI division directors on extramural scientific research program policy, progress, and future direction of programs within each division. This includes evaluating NCI awarded grants, cooperative agreements, contracts, and merit review of concepts and activities consistent with the Institute's programs.
- The advisory role is scientific and does not include deliberation on matters of public policy.
- Examines the extramural programs and their infrastructures to evaluate whether changes are necessary to ensure the Institute is positioned to effectively guide and administer the needs of science research in the foreseeable future.

Three times a year[b]

- Advises the directors of the Intramural Division of NCI and the NCI director and deputy director on NCI's intramural scientific program policy, progress, and the future direction of the research programs of each division. Includes performance and productivity evaluation of each division and of staff scientists through site visits to intramural laboratories. The advisory role of the Board is scientific and does not include deliberation on matters of public policy.

Three times a year[b]

Advises and make recommendations to the NCI director for oversight and integration of the planning and advisory groups serving the programmatic and institutional objectives of the Institute. Serves as the official channel through which the findings and recommendations emerging from these groups are submitted to NCI. They consider the reports of the various review groups as informational, as advisory, or as recommendations, and assist NCI in identifying research opportunities or needs within areas of cancer research that cut across the intramural and extramural programs.

Biannual

(continued on next page)

TABLE 4-2   *continued*

Name	Structure
	• NCI advisory committee to the director
	• Three nonvoting ex officio members
	Members serve for the duration of their terms of their respective boards.
NCI Initial Review Group	Number of appointees varies. Members are authorities knowledgeable in the various disciplines and fields related to scientific areas relevant to NCI's programs. The permanent membership may be supplemented at any meeting through temporary appointments of specific scientists whose expertise is necessary to review grant applications under consideration at that meeting. Members appointed by the NCI director serve 4-year terms.
NCI Special Emphasis Group (SEP), established by NCI director September 1995	Approximately 660 reviewers serve each year and are outstanding authorities in various fields of biomedical research. Members and chairs are not formally appointed, but serve for individual meetings on an as-needed basis in response to specific applications, proposals, or proposed solicitations under review.
Director's Consumer Liaison Group[a]	15 appointed members who are consumer advocates involved in cancer advocacy and represent a constituency with which they communicate on a regular basis. Appointed by the NCI director to serve 3-year terms.

[a] These advisory groups are unique to NCI. Because of its unique congressional charter and substantial funding, NCI plays a special role in research that is sponsored by NIH. To support its extensive research programs, NCI uses additional advisory committees that carry special responsibilities. The President's Cancer Panel and the National Cancer Advisory Board are the only two advisory groups at NIH whose members are all appointed by the President. They have oversight over all NCI activities, and ensure that NCI programs maintain goals focused on the nation's interests and needs in cancer. To provide additional cohesion, communication, and

Function	Meetings
The IRG, made up of seven specialized subcommittees, reviews and advises the NCI director and the director of NCI's Division of Extramural Activities on the scientific and technical merit of applications and proposals for research grants, research training grants, cooperative agreements and cancer centers, and contract proposals relating to scientific areas associated with all facets of cancer.	Three times a year[b]
Reviews grant proposals, cooperative agreement applications, contract proposals for research projects, and applications for research and training activities in broad areas of basic and clinical cancer research. Advises the NCI director and the director of NCI's Division of Extramural Activities regarding research grant and cooperative agreement applications, contract proposals, and concept review relating to basic and clinical sciences and applied R&D programs.	Held as necessary —about 60 per year
Provides advice and makes recommendations to the NCI director from the perspective and viewpoint of cancer consumer advocate, on a wide variety of issues, programs, and research priorities. Also serves as a channel for consumer advocates to voice their views and concerns.	Biannual[b]

management across all NCI activities, an advisory committee to the director was formed, with members representing all NCI program advisory and oversight groups. Finally, recognizing the important and influential role of the cancer advocacy community, NCI organized a Consumer's Liaison Group to ensure interaction and communication between the advocacy population and the cancer research community.

[b]All meetings are open to the public unless otherwise noted.
SOURCE: <http://deainfo.nci.nih.gov/ADVISORY/boards.htm>.

> ## BOX 4-4   Categories of the National Cancer Institute's Major Budget Activities
>
> **Cancer Causation Research:** Studies the events involved in the initiation and promotion of cancer. It encompasses chemical and physical carcinogenesis, biological carcinogenesis, epidemiology, chemoprevention, and nutrition research. Studies focus on external agents such as chemicals; radiation; fibers and other particles; viruses; parasitic infections; and host factors such as hormone levels, nutritional and immunologic status, and the genetic composition of the individual (approximately 30 percent of the NCI budget in 1997).
>
> **Detection and Diagnosis Research:** Includes studies to improve diagnostic accuracy, provide better prognostic information to guide therapeutic decisions, monitor the response to therapy more effectively, detect cancer at its earliest presentation, and identify populations and individuals at increased risk for the development of cancer (approximately 6 percent of the NCI budget in 1997).
>
> **Treatment Research:** Includes preclinical and clinical research. Preclinical research focuses on the discovery of new antitumor agents and their development in preparation for testing in clinical trials. These agents include both synthetic compounds and natural products. Clinical research involves demonstrating the effectiveness of new anticancer treatments through their systematic testing in clinical trials (Phases I, II, and III) (approximately 30 percent of the NCI budget in 1997).
>
> **Cancer Biology Research:** Encompasses basic research on cancer and the body's response to cancer. Studies include investigations of cellular and molecular characteristics of tumor cells, interactions between cells within a tumor, and the components of the host immune defense mechanisms. The ultimate goal is to identify and explain the stepwise progression between the initiating event in the cell and final tumor development (approximately 15 percent of the NCI budget in 1997).
>
> **Resource Development:** Includes support for the Cancer Centers Program (7 percent of the NCI budget in 1997), training and career development awards (approximately 3.5 percent of the budget), and construction (approximately 0.1 percent of the budget).
>
> **Cancer Prevention and Control:** Includes basic and applied research through both intramural and extramural mechanisms in all phases of cancer prevention and control, as well as cancer surveillance. A key priority of the program is to develop strategies for the effective translation of knowledge gained from prevention and control research into health promotion and disease prevention activities for the benefit of the public (approximately 10 percent of the NCI budget in 1997).
>
> ---
>
> SOURCE: "The NCI Grants Process, Part III: Funding Allocations and Mechanisms." See <http://www.nci.nih.gov/admin/gab/98GPB/98GPBp3.htm>.

program initiatives; program priorities; previous commitments, such as noncompeting continuations; and other projected needs. Extramural research is funded by NIH through three major mechanisms—grants, cooperative agreements, and contracts (see Box 4-5). Approval of a project may include a recommendation for support for up to 5 years. Because awards

---

BOX 4-5   Mechanisms of Financial Support through the National Institutes of Health

Grants: Used when (1) no substantial programmatic involvement is anticipated between NCI and the recipient during performance of the financially assisted activities, thus allowing the recipient freedom of action in carrying out the research project; and (2) NCI has no expectation of a specified service or end product for its use.

Cooperative Agreements: Used (1) when the applicant is responding to a specific NCI announcement for cooperative agreements and must tailor the proposal to its requirements; (2) when substantial programmatic involvement is anticipated between NCI and the recipient during the performance of the activities; and (3) generally, for any new or competing continuation R01 investigator-initiated clinical trial, prevention or control intervention, or epidemiological study in which direct costs exceed $500,000 in any year.

Contracts: Used to acquire cancer research and developmental efforts and other resources or services needed by the federal government from other organizations. Projects are conducted with the direct involvement of NCI. In contrast to assistance mechanisms, which are used to support and stimulate research, contracts (procurement) are used when the principal purpose of the transaction is to acquire a specific service or end product for the direct benefit of or use by NCI.

SOURCE: "The NCI Grants Process, Part I: An Overview." See <http://www.nci.nih.gov/admin/gab/98GPB/98GPBp1.htm>.

---

are subject to the appropriation of funds by Congress each year, however, they are generally made on an annual basis, with the exception of a few unique programs. For each additional year within the project period, the principal investigator must request funds through a noncompeting continuation application, in which scientific progress may be taken into consideration.[7]

NIH Peer Review of Funding Applications

Peer review of NIH research grant applications was formally mandated in 1974 by Section 475 of the Public Health Service Act, although the tradition and system of peer review had already been in place for many years. Three peer review cycles or "rounds" per year are offered. NIH funding may be sought by nonprofit and for-profit organizations, institutions of higher education, hospitals, research foundations, governments

---

[7] "The NCI Grants Process, Part II: Process and Administration"; see <http://www.nci.nih.gov/admin/gab/98GPB/98GPBp2.htm>.

and their agencies, and, occasionally, individuals.[8] Most applications are unsolicited and are initiated by the principal investigator. As a result, each application received must be assigned by NIH staff to the most appropriate review group and funding Institute when it arrives at NIH.

There are two levels of review for applications submitted to NIH (see Box 4-2). The NIH Center for Scientific Review (CSR) provides oversight of the initial peer review process and also assigns applications to specific NIH Institutes and Centers in the event that they are recommended for funding. Integrated review groups (IRGs), whose primary function is to review and evaluate the scientific merit of research grant applications, perform the first level of review. Nineteen chartered IRGs distributed among three review divisions[9] within CSR review applications regardless of the NIH Institute assignment. In the past, the roughly 100 study sections were arrayed under the 19 IRGs according to scientific discipline (e.g., cell biology, pathology, biochemistry, bacteriology), but there is currently a move to reorganize the study sections into groups that are more problem or disease oriented. Generally, an IRG study section is composed of 12 to 18 mainly nonfederal scientists who are selected on the basis of their recognized expertise in their respective research fields. During each of the three cycles, a CSR IRG study section may review between 50 and 100 grant applications.[10] Because grants are generally funded in the order of their rating relative to other applications in the same field, the fact that a study section has been constituted in a particular area of science usually guarantees that at least some applications in that area will be funded. As a result, the NIH attempts to monitor changes occurring in science to ensure that study sections, as a group, are appropriately constituted to assess the research applications in all areas of scientific endeavor. The creation of new study sections, the restructuring of established study sections, and the use of special panels can have a significant impact on the areas of science funded by NIH. Thus, any proposed changes in the study sections are carefully considered.[11]

The individual Institutes and Centers may also establish their own IRGs to review special types of basic and clinical research and education or training grant applications. For example, NCI has its own IRGs to

---

[8] Foreign institutions and international organizations are eligible to receive only research grants.

[9] The three review divisions are the Division of Cellular and Molecular Mechanisms, Division of Physiological Systems, and Division of Clinical and Population-Based Studies.

[10] "The NCI Grants Process, Part II: Process and Administration." See also the website for the Center Scientific Review: <http://www.drg.nih.gov/review/peerrev.htm>.

[11] "Setting Research Priorities at the National Institutes of Health"; <http://www.nih.gov/news/ResPriority/priority.htm#Funds>.

review applications for program project grants, cancer center support grants, clinical trials, cooperative group agreements, training grants for graduate and postdoctoral fellows, and cancer education grants. Many of the applications reviewed by NCI-specific IRGs must undergo project site visits because of their specialized and complex nature. In contrast, only about 1 percent of the research grant applications reviewed by the CSR require a site visit before the IRG can complete its assessment. For any applications referred to NCI for review that cannot be reviewed by an IRG for reasons of conflict of interest or lack of expertise, special emphasis panels (SEPs) (formerly special review committees [SRCs]) are assembled for the review.

Once the first level of review has been completed, a second level of review is undertaken within each of the individual Institutes and Centers. For grants referred to NCI, the second level of review, which was mandated by the National Cancer Institute Act in 1937 and incorporated into the Public Health Service Act in 1944, is performed by the National Cancer Advisory Board (NCAB).[12] The NCAB is responsible for the final external review of all grant applications, except those requesting $50,000 or less in direct costs per year, individual fellowship applications, applications with percentiles in the bottom one-half of those reviewed by the CSR, and applications not recommended for further consideration. The NCAB's responsibility is to evaluate all grant applications in relation to the needs of NCI and the priorities of the National Cancer Program. In most cases, the NCAB concurs with the IRG recommendations.

In 1997, NIH appointed a committee[13] to examine the process by which scientific review groups rate grant applications and to propose recommendations for improving that process in light of scientific knowledge of measurement and decision making. The committee's charge was formulated in response to the perception that the review of grant applications needed to focus more on the quality of the science and the impact it might have on the field than on the details of technique and methodology. As a result, reviewers are now instructed to address five specific review criteria: the importance of the problem or question, the innovation employed in approaching the problem, the adequacy of the methodology proposed, the qualifications and experience of the investigator, and the scientific environment in which the work will be done (see Box 4-6). Reviewers then assign a single, global score for each scored application. This

---

[12] The NCAB is composed of 18 members who are appointed by the President. Members serve overlapping terms of 6 years.

[13] The Rating of Grant Applications subcommittee of the NIH Committee on Improving Peer Review.

**BOX 4-6　Specific Criteria for NIH Peer Review of
Grant Applications**

Significance: Does this study address an important problem? If the aims of the application are achieved, how will scientific knowledge be advanced? What will be the effect of these studies on the concepts or methods that drive this field?

Approach: Are the conceptual framework, design, methods, and analyses adequately developed, well integrated, and appropriate to the aims of the project? Does the applicant acknowledge potential problem areas and consider alternative tactics?

Innovation: Does the project employ novel concepts, approaches, or methods? Are the aims original and innovative? Does the project challenge existing paradigms or develop new methodologies or technologies?

Investigator: Is the investigator appropriately trained and well suited to carry out this work? Is the work proposed appropriate to the experience level of the principal investigator and other researchers (if any)?

Environment: Does the scientific environment in which the work will be done contribute to the probability of success? Do the proposed experiments take advantage of unique features of the scientific environment or employ useful collaborative arrangements? Is there evidence of institutional support?

SOURCE: *Review Criteria for the Rating of Unsolicited Research Grant and Other Applications,* NIH Guide, Volume 26, Number 22, June 27, 1997 (<http://grants.nih.gov/grants/guide/notice-files/not97-010.html>).

---

score is intended to reflect the project's potential overall impact on the field based on consideration of the five criteria, with the emphasis on each criterion varying from one application to another, depending on the nature of the application and its relative strengths. In other words, an application does not need to be strong in all categories to be judged likely to have a major scientific impact and thus deserve a high-priority score.[14]

While these review criteria are intended for use primarily with unsolicited research project applications (e.g., R01, P01), they also provide a starting point for review of solicited applications and nonresearch activities. However, solicited applications must also address additional specific criteria for scientific peer review. Because many perceive a bias against unorthodox research in the NIH peer review process (Wessely and Wood, 1999; Gillespie et al., 1985), the solicitation of applications, with specific review criteria, may be critical for funding large-scale projects through NIH, as discussed further below. Equally important is how decisions are

---

[14] *Review Criteria for the Rating of Unsolicited Research Grant and Other Applications,* NIH Guide, Volume 26, Number 22, June 27, 1997 (<http://grants.nih.gov/grants/guide/notice-files/not97-010.html>).

made to solicit and review applications in novel areas (for example, with input from leaders in the field as well as NIH staff).

Several challenges associated with peer review may be particularly difficult for large-scale projects.[15] For example, avoiding conflict of interest on the review panel may be exceptionally problematical in the case of large-scale projects. If most of the experts in a particular area of investigation are included in a consortium or network (or in competing applications for consortia), it may be difficult to find reviewers with appropriate expertise. Moreover, those who are not included in a consortium could potentially be resentful and therefore not objective. In addition, some reviewers may disagree with the need for a large-scale approach and thus be tempted to review the concept of large-scale research rather than the scientific and technical merits of specific proposals.

Funding Mechanisms for Extramural Research and Solicitation of NIH Grant Applications

NIH has many different mechanisms for funding extramural research. Examples of those that are most relevant to a discussion of large-scale science are shown in Box 4-7. As noted above, the majority of grant applications to NIH are unsolicited. The most common mechanism for funding investigator-initiated research proposals is the R01 research project grant, often referred to as a traditional research grant. In 1999, there were 22,000 such grants with an average award size of $275,000. A somewhat related mechanism is the P01 program project grant, which provides funding for multiple independent investigators who are studying a similar topic using common resources. Given the average size of these grants, however, the traditional, unsolicited mechanism of extramural funding is not very amenable to large-scale projects.

Perhaps one of the greatest impediments to obtaining funding for large-scale projects through the traditional approach are the restrictions NIH places on grant applications that request funds for direct costs in excess of $500,000 per year. Such applications are accepted for review and consideration only if the applicants have obtained an agreement to do so from Institute or Center staff at least 6 weeks prior to the anticipated submission.[16] This policy pertains to all unsolicited applications, includ-

---

[15]Arthur Zachary, Scientific Review Administrator at the National Institute of General Medical Sciences, in a presentation at an NIH forum on administrative strategies entitled "Big Science, Big Challenges," Bethesda, MD, March 1, 2002.

[16]NIH Notice for Acceptance for review of unsolicited applications that request more than $500,000 in direct costs, effective June 1, 1998; see <http://grants.nih.gov/grants/guide/notice-files/not98-030.html>. Notice updated October 16, 2001; see <http://grants.nih.gov/grants/guide/notice-files/NOT-OD-02-004.html>.

BOX 4-7   Examples of NIH Funding Mechanisms for Investigator-Initiated Research Grants

R01 Research Project Grant: Supports a discrete, specified research project to be performed by the named investigator in an area representing his/her specific interests and competencies. This is generally referred to as a traditional research project.

P01 Program Project Grant: Supports an integrated, multiproject research approach involving a number of independent investigators who share knowledge and common resources. This type of grant has a defined central research focus involving several disciplines or several aspects of one discipline. Each individual project must contribute to or be directly related to the common theme of the total research effort, thus forming a system of research activities and projects directed toward a well-defined research program goal.

P50 Specialized Center Grant: Supports any part of the full range of research and development, from very basic to clinical activities. The spectrum of activities forms a multidisciplinary attack on cancer. These grants differ from Program Project Grants in that they are usually developed in response to an announcement of the programmatic needs of NCI and later receive continuous attention from its staff. Centers may also serve as regional or national resources for special research purposes.

U01 Cooperative Agreement: Supports a discrete, specified, circumscribed project to be performed by the named investigator(s) in an area representing their specific interests and competencies. This mechanism is used when substantial programmatic involvement is anticipated between NCI and the recipient during performance of the contemplated activity.

U19 Research Program Cooperative Agreement: Supports a research program of multiple projects directed toward a specific major objective, basic theme, or program goal, requiring a broadly based multidisciplinary and often long-term approach. Substantial federal programmatic staff involvement is intended to assist investigators during the performance of research activities, as defined in the terms and conditions of the award. This mechanism can provide support for certain basic shared resources, including clinical components, which facilitate the total research effort.

U24 Resource-Related Research Project Cooperative Agreement: Supports research projects that contribute to improving the capability of resources to serve biomedical research.

U54 Specialized Center Cooperative Agreements: Supports any part of the full range of research and development, from very basic to clinical; may involve ancillary supportive activities, such as protracted patient care, necessary to the primary research or research and development effort. The spectrum of activities forms a multidisciplinary attack on a specific disease entity or biomedical problem area. These efforts differ from program projects in that they are usually developed in response to an announcement of the programmatic needs of an Institute or division and subsequently receive continuous attention from its staff. Centers may also serve as regional or national resources for special research purposes.

BOX 4-7 *continued*

R21 Exploratory/Developmental Grant: Pilot grants support the development of new research activities in categorical program areas, a common mechanism for technology development.

R33 Exploratory/Developmental Grant—Phase II: Provides a second phase with a larger budget for the support of innovative, exploratory, and developmental research activities initiated under the R21 mechanism.

SOURCE: "The NCI Grants Process, Part III: Funding Allocations and Mechanisms." See <http://www.nci.nih.gov/admin/gab/98GPB/98GPBp3.htm>.

ing new applications, competing continuations, competing supplements, and any amended version of a previous grant application. Although NIH can and does support some research projects with large budgets, the policy states that unanticipated requests for unusually high amounts of direct costs, despite the merit of the application and the justification for the budget, are difficult to manage by NIH staff. Thus, the Institute needs to consider the possibility of such awards as early as possible in the budget and program planning process.

However, this policy does not apply to applications submitted in response to NIH program announcements (PAs) or requests for applications (RFAs), which include their own specific budgetary limits. PAs and RFAs are used by NIH to encourage the submission of grant applications in a particular topic or field of research in order to stimulate new, expanded, or high-priority programs. PAs describe continuing, new, or expanded program interests for which funding applications are invited. Applications in response to PAs are generally reviewed through the CSR, similar to the process for unsolicited grant applications. Funds for PAs may or may not be set aside, so this is the simplest form of "special attention" to indicate NIH interest. Some programs operate for years under a standing PA. The RFA is a more assertive method—an invitation to submit grant proposals in a well-defined scientific area to stimulate activity in priority programs. An RFA has a target budget with earmarked funds and specific closing dates for applications, and review is usually handled by Institutes themselves, rather than the CSR. Contracts have a similar mechanism—the request for proposals.

Many PAs and RFAs use cooperative agreements such as the U01, U19, U24, and U54 as a funding mechanism. As noted in Box 4-5, cooperative agreements require applicants to tailor their proposals in response to specific NCI announcements, and involve substantial programmatic involvement and oversight by NCI staff during the performance of the research. This mechanism is also used for investigator-initiated clinical trials, prevention or control interventions, or epidemiological studies in which direct costs exceed $500,000 per year. Because of these characteristics, cooperative agreements may offer more flexibility in defining nontraditional goals and end products of the research, and thus could ease the peer review process for large-scale projects. Peer review of NIH grants has always emphasized hypothesis-driven research, and reviewers have disparaged projects designed to generate large classes of data that would fit the operational definition of large-scale science in this report as "fishing expeditions." This obstacle might be overcome by defining the criteria for proposals in an RFA.

Solicited applications may also use the two-phased R21 (phase I) and R33 (phase II) grant mechanism (see Box 4-5). These awards, known as exploratory/developmental grants, are used to support the development of new research activities in a short pilot phase (R21, up to $100,000/year for 6 months to 2 years) and a longer follow-up development phase (R33, generally up to $500,000/year for 4 years). As such, these grants are highly amenable to non–hypothesis-driven research focused on the development of new technologies, including research performed by or in collaboration with industry.[17] The purpose of the grants, which are usually awarded as an R21/R33 combination, is to stimulate exploration of new, high-risk, biomedical technology research and development that will generate preliminary data to support a future application for a NIH R01 grant. For both the R21 and R33, there are definite milestones and deliverables built into the grant language that must be met. An R33 could become immediately available to an R21 grantee when predefined project milestones have been achieved. The phase I/phase II combination award could provide up to five years of funding to develop new or improved instruments, technologies, or computer software. At that point, it is assumed that the technologies will have matured enough for the investigator to compete for a follow-on award through another grant mechanism, usually an R01.[18] Because this mechanism is used for the development of new initiatives, it does not provide for long-term support on a large scale. Thus, investigators must eventually convert successful research programs to more conventional NIH funding mechanisms, which can be risky and lead to delays or loss of funding. For example, if a follow-up grant application has to be submitted as an R01, it will be reviewed as a new application and the IRG committee reviewing it for the first time may be completely unaware of the history of NCI support for the project, the reason for supporting

---

[17] See <http://otir.nci.nih.gov/index.html>.
[18] Communication with Edward Monachino, NCI Office of Technology and Industrial Relations, August 20, 2002.

development of the technology in the first place, or the interest from NCI in continuing the application of the technology. This may be especially problematic if application of the technology does not fit with the IRG reviewer's expectation of hypothesis-driven research. Furthermore, budgets in some of these grant applications tend to be large and this also may raise questions in a review panel that is accustomed to reviewing traditional R01 applications with smaller budgets.

Given the power and flexibility of the PA and RFA mechanisms for the solicitation of funding applications, decisions to issue them can be very influential in defining new goals and priorities within NIH. But there is no Institute-wide policy for this decision-making process. Extramural program directors are charged with "reviewing and evaluating the state of the art of research in a specific program area and stimulating scientific investigations in that field through the issuance of RFAs and PAs."[19] How this is accomplished varies greatly across and within Institutes and Centers, however, and may change over time. For example, ideas may be suggested by a variety of sources, including outside advisory, review, or working groups; division and Institute directors; and individual scientists. Discussions regarding a potential solicitation generally take place within a division, but often include people from outside the division as well. If a concept has been formally approved within the originating division, it goes on to be reviewed by the Institute's executive committee, which can either approve it, send it back for revisions, or reject it. The concept may then be formally presented at an open meeting of the Board of Scientific Advisors for consideration.[20] This approach was used by NCI to launch several large-scale initiatives, including the Cancer Genome Anatomy Project (CGAP), the Early Detection Research Network (EDRN), and the Specialized Programs of Research Excellence (SPORE) grant program. Such an ad hoc approach to generating new solicitations for applications can inhibit rapid action on promising new initiatives, especially since the application and review process can take an additional year from the time the solicitation is formally announced.

Recently, NCI solicited suggestions for new initiatives through the Office of Scientific Opportunities. Specifically, the agency sought ideas for "extraordinary opportunities"[21] that:

- Respond to important recent developments in knowledge and technology.

---

[19] "The NCI Grants Process, Part II: Process and Administration."

[20] Personal communication, Robert E. Wittes, former NCI deputy director, Office of Extramural Science, and director, Division of Cancer Treatment and Diagnosis.

[21] NCI Office of Scientific Opportunities; see <http://cancer.gov/oso/extrord.htm>.

- Offer approaches to cancer research that go beyond the size, scope, and funding of NCI's current research activities.
- Can be implemented with specific, defined investments.
- Can be described in terms of achievable milestones, with clear consequences for not investing.
- Promise advances that are needed for making progress against all cancers.

Both PAs and RFAs have been used previously to launch large-scale projects within NIH. For example, they have been used to initiate some of the models of large-scale science described in Chapter 3, including the National Institute of General Medical Sciences (NIGMS) Protein Structure Initiative and Large-Scale Collaborative Projects, as well as the NCI Mouse Models of Human Cancer Consortium. In the case of the HGP, a further step was taken in creating a new Institute. That level of support, which requires action by the authorizing committees in both houses of Congress, is not likely to be repeated for the types of large-scale projects described in this report. Once an Institute has been created, it is unlikely to be dismantled,[22] so questions have been posed regarding the future activities of the NHGRI once its primary goal of sequencing the human genome has been achieved (Pennisi, 2002). Currently, the Institute is focusing on sequencing the genomes of other species, but some have suggested that it should branch out into related areas, such as structural biology and proteomics, to ensure its long-term relevance and survival. Furthermore, the number of institutes within NIH has increased from 7 to 24 in the last 40 years, and this growth has been strongly criticized by former NIH director Harold Varmus and others on the grounds of the associated loss of flexibility, managerial capacity, and coordination, and the accompanying increase in administrative burden (Varmus, 2001). Several former leaders from NIH have argued that giving the NIH director more power over Institute policy and budgets would facilitate cross-institutional programs in such fields as genomics and bioinformatics (Metheny, 2002). The structure and organization of NIH are the focus of an ongoing NRC study.[23]

There are a number of ways in which temporary infrastructures could be established for the purpose of conducting a large-scale biomedical research project. For example, leasing space would make it easier to

---

[22] NIH is somewhat unusual in that its initial authorization (Public Health Service Act of 1944) does not require reauthorization.

[23] The study, Organizational Structure of NIH, will examine such topics as budgets, management processes, peer review, and authorities for and functions of councils and committees. See <http://www4.nationalacademies.org/cp.nsf>.

downsize a project upon completion of its research goals. Likewise, phase out funding could enable investigators to reduce their research efforts on a particular project over the course of 2–3 years.

NONFEDERAL FUNDING OF LARGE-SCALE BIOMEDICAL RESEARCH PROJECTS

Although the federal government is the largest single funder of biomedical research, there are many other groups that sponsor research as well, including industry, philanthropies, and other nonprofit organizations. But it can be more difficult to quantify and characterize these sources. For example, NCI is still the largest single provider of funds for cancer research, but other NIH Institutes and federal agencies, as well as many other organizations—including pharmaceutical and biotechnology companies and nonprofit organizations—now contribute about half of the total (McGeary and Burstein, 1999). The various contributions are difficult to define precisely because the relevance of some research to cancer is not easily identified or predicted. The challenge is even greater when one is attempting to quantify the amount of funding allocated for large-scale projects by the various funding sectors. The variability in the definition of large-scale science is an obstacle in itself, further complicated by additional variability in the reporting and public disclosure of funding allocations among the different nonfederal sources.

A study by the Global Forum for Health Research,[24] published in 2001, can shed some light on the funding sources for biomedical R&D in more general terms (see Table 4-3). Worldwide, public funding in 1998 accounted for 50 percent of all support for biomedical research, and 57 percent of that portion came from the United States. In other words, about one-quarter of all funding for biomedical R&D worldwide came from public U.S sources. Private industry provided another 42 percent, while nonprofit organizations contributed 8 percent of the total. About 50 percent of the nonprofit funding also originated in the United States. The two largest private, nonprofit sponsors of biomedical research in 1998 were the Wellcome Trust in the United Kingdom ($650 million for biomedical research) and the Howard Hughes Medical Institute (HHMI) in the United States ($389 million). It is not possible to provide a breakdown of the global industry total by country, in large part because the majority of pharmaceutical research is funded by multinational companies. However, the study cites national sources indicating that pharmaceutical and biotechnology companies in the United States invested $20.3 billion in

---

[24] See <http://www.globalforumhealth.org>.

TABLE 4-3   Estimated Global Health R&D Funding in 1998

Source	Estimated Total for 1998[a]	%
Public funding	37.0	50
Private industry funding	30.5	42
Nonprofit funding	6.0	8
Total	73.5	100

[a] Billions of current $US.
SOURCE: Adapted from: The Global Forum for Health Research, 2001.

biomedical R&D (two-thirds of the industry total), with $16.9 billion spent at home and $3.4 billion abroad.

For academic research in the United States, the federal government provided the lion's share of funding—almost 60 percent in 2000 (see Figure 4-2). Another 20 percent was provided by academic institutions themselves. Industry accounted for an estimated 8 percent of academic R&D in 2000, while 7 percent came from state and local governments. The remaining funds (about 7 percent) came from a variety of sources, including nonprofits, voluntary health agencies, and gifts from individuals (National Science Foundation, 2002).

Industry Funding of Large-Scale Biomedical Research

Industry can contribute to biomedical research in many different ways. The most common is for a company to maintain its own R&D programs. In recent years, it has also become more common for companies to establish collaborations with academic scientists or institutions, or to provide direct funding for projects undertaken by scientists in academia. In the latter case, this funding may be the sole support for a project, or it may complement funding provided by federal or other sources. This shift is likely due in part to passage of the Bayh-Dole act, which allows academic institutions to retain patent rights to discoveries made using federal funds (discussed in greater detail in Chapter 7). Often, scientists seek industry funding for projects that are less likely to be funded by NIH because they are risky, very costly, or simply do not fit within NIH's current funding mechanisms or priorities. Once such projects have been established or pilot projects have demonstrated proof of principle, however, scientists are more likely to seek and obtain federal funding. Thus, industry can spur novel research directions or fill gaps left by federal funding. An example of such a scenario is described in Box 4-8. However, some large funding agreements between academia and industry have been scaled back or eliminated recently, leading some to speculate that such agreements are less likely to be initiated in the future (Lawler, 2003).

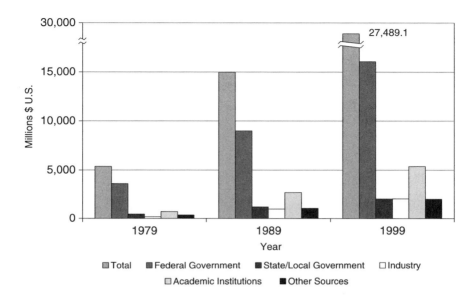

FIGURE 4-2 Sources of academic R&D funds: 1979, 1989, 1999.
SOURCE: National Science Foundation, 2002, Appendix Table 5-3.

Companies have also contributed by establishing nonprofit entities that produce data for public use and dissemination. Merck has made several such contributions in recent years. For example, it established the Merck Genome Research Institute to identify expressed sequence tags and to place them in a publicly accessible database in collaboration with NHGRI and NCI. This initiative was undertaken to prevent private institutions, such as Human Genome Sciences, from retaining patent rights to all expressed sequence tags (ESTs). This effort also provided inspiration for the SNP Consortium, a public–private collaboration to identify and disseminate genetic polymorphisms (described in Chapter 3).

A recent survey[25] of worldwide funding for genomics may be relevant to the discussion of large-scale biomedical research funding by industry in particular. Although not all research in the field of genomics qualifies as large-scale science as defined in this report, a significant portion is likely devoted to such projects, and thus these data may offer some

---

[25] World Survey of Funding for Genomics Research; see <http://www.stanford.edu/class/siw198q/websites/genomics/entry.htm>.

BOX 4-8   Example of a Large-Scale Project Launched with Funding from Philanthropy and Industry

In the early 1990s, Dr. Nancy Hopkins, professor of biology at the Massachusetts Institute of Technology (MIT), began to propose a novel approach for identifying important developmental genes in zebra fish, a laboratory model commonly used to study development. The standard approach for finding genes in this model was chemical mutagenesis followed by positional cloning—a very laborious undertaking for each gene of interest. Dr. Hopkins decided to address this problem using a retrovirus to generate insertional mutations that could then be easily amplified to identify the target gene.

Initially, the project was viewed as very risky because this approach had never been used in zebra fish, and there were many technical difficulties to overcome. The project was begun with a small amount of philanthropic funding at MIT. Dr. Hopkins then applied for National Science Foundation funding, and following a site visit, she was awarded a small grant. She also applied for NIH funding, but the project was viewed as too risky, in part because of the technical obstacles noted above and in part because she was new to the zebra fish field.

Dr. Hopkins then identified a viral vector that would insert efficiently and randomly into the fish genome, and also could be grown to high titer. About the same time, Amgen provided MIT with $20 million for research. MIT investigators wrote proposals, and a committee selected several to send to officials at Amgen, who then made the final choice. Dr. Hopkins received enough funding to do a pilot study, which demonstrated that the method could work. When she then reapplied for NIH funding, the project was seen as posing a much lower risk, and she was awarded a grant for $500,000. Amgen provided another $700,000 so she could do a full screen of the genome. With this combined funding, her laboratory has cloned 300 genes involved in development; this is in contrast to approximately 70 genes that have been identified and cloned by the rest of the field using chemical mutagenesis. Dr. Hopkins estimates that the cost per gene using her approach was about 5 to 10 percent that of the traditional method.

---

relevant insight. In the year 2000, private industry spent more on genomic research than all governments and nonprofit groups combined (see Figure 4-3). Indeed, the largest portion of funding was derived from companies identified as "genomics firms." These companies are devoted exclusively to genomics research, and thus could be construed as private ventures in large-scale science. More than 70 percent of these 270 companies, both publicly traded and privately held firms, are based in the United States. The dramatic growth in the number of these firms in recent years and the rapid increase in their market value (see Figure 4-4) suggest that this may be an effective approach to large-scale genomics research. However, the long-term success and viability of these ventures, which are all relatively new, remain to be demonstrated. Furthermore, many questions have been raised regarding intellectual property issues associated with

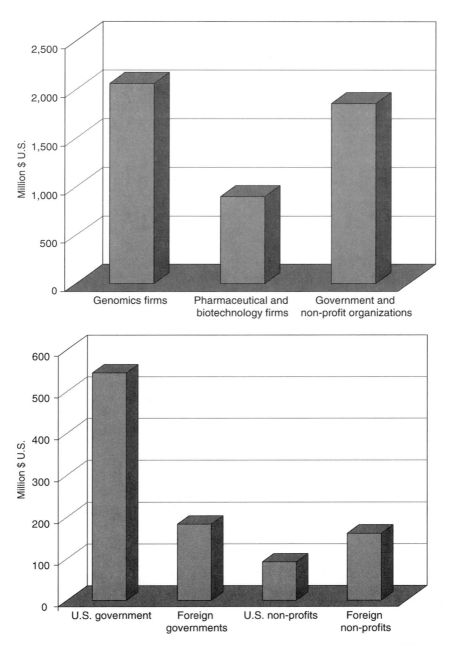

FIGURE 4-3 Worldwide funding for genomics research, 2000 (millions of $U.S.).
SOURCE: World Survey of Funding for Genomics and Stanford in Washington
Program, http://www.stanford.edu/class/siw198q/websites/genomics.

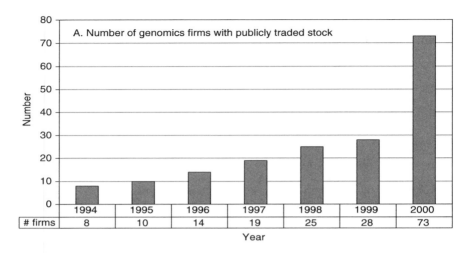

# firms	8	10	14	19	25	28	73

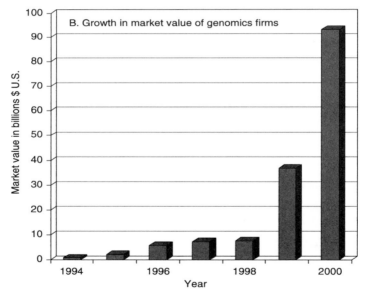

FIGURE 4-4   Growth of commercial genomics. A: Number of firms with publicly traded stock. B: Growth in market value of genomics firms.
SOURCE: World Survey of Funding for Genomics, Stanford in Washington Program, http://www.stanford.edu/class/siw198q/websites/genomics.

large-scale projects undertaken solely in the private sector, as is discussed further in Chapter 7.

These very concerns recently led to a unique public–private collaboration to sequence the mouse genome. NHGRI began a mouse sequencing project in 1999 by providing funding to 10 laboratories using a combination of sequencing strategies, such as sequencing randomly chosen DNA or particular DNA regions of biological interest. In the spring of 2000, the publicly funded group chose to a adopt a hybrid strategy—combining data generated by the whole-genome shotgun approach for most of the genome with some sequences generated the more traditional way, using genomic maps. This decision was based on the success of the *Drosophila* sequencing project[26] and on pilot projects conducted by the mouse sequencers (Pennisi, 2000b). Shortly thereafter, Celera began sequencing the genomes of three different strains of laboratory mice on its own. Within 6 months, Celera was offering access to a database of these sequences to anyone willing and able to pay a user fee. Because of a strong desire at NIH and in the research community to have a sequence that was freely available to the public, a new public–private consortium was announced in the fall of 2000, with the goal of sequencing the genome of a fourth mouse strain (Marshall, 2000). Six Institutes at NIH, including NCI, two companies, and two nonprofit organizations provided $58 million to sequence the genome in 6 months using the whole-genome shotgun approach employed by Celera. The new money was divided among only three sequencing centers—two in the United States and one in the United Kingdom—to complete the work. On May 6, 2002, the Mouse Genome Sequencing Consortium announced the completion of a draft sequence for one common laboratory strain of mouse, which is available free of charge through the Internet (Marshall, 2002b). In fact, the consortium released data in real time to a public database throughout the project, with no restrictions. However, the public project was criticized initially for not making a greater effort to assemble the mouse genome sequences into a form that would enable the study of gene structure and function (Marshall, 2001).

A less competitive approach was subsequently taken in sequencing the rat genome through a public–private consortium. That project, which is also using a strategy that combines a map-based sequencing approach and Celera's whole-genome shotgun approach, is funded jointly by NHGRI and the National Heart, Lung, and Blood Institute (NHLBI) (Marshall, 2001; Hafner, 2001). In this case, however, a substantial fraction ($21 million out

---

[26] In the case of the *Drosophila* genome, a group of NHGRI-funded researchers supplied Celera with more than 10,000 cloned fragments of DNA to which the company applied the shotgun sequencing method. The data were released to the public (Pennisi, 1999).

of a $58 million total) of the most recent batch of NIH funding will go to Celera to perform the sequencing. Much of the remaining funding will go to a second sequencing company, Genome Therapeutics Corporation. Because the funding is derived from federal sources, the participants agreed to abide by a set of mandatory data-release rules that require grantees to publicly release raw sequence data on a weekly basis. This approach may be a model for future endeavors. While avoiding duplication of public and private efforts, it provides a cost-effective mechanism for producing a public good (a freely available sequence database) using industry standards for staffing, management, and quality control.

Another approach to establishing public–private collaborations is a cooperative research and development agreement (CRADA). Under the Federal Technology Transfer Act (FTTA) of 1986, federal agencies have been mandated to encourage and facilitate collaboration among federal laboratories, state and local governments, universities, and the private sector in order to assist in the transfer of federal technology to the market place. One vehicle for this collaboration is through a CRADA. Examples of products that have resulted in part through a CRADA include Havrix® and Taxol®.

A CRADA is a contractual agreement[27] between one or more federal laboratories and one or more industrial or university partners, under which the federal laboratories provide personnel, services, facilities, equipment, or other resources with or without reimbursement and the nonfederal parties provide funds, personnel, services, facilities, equipment, or other resources toward the conduct of a particular R&D program. The purpose of a CRADA is to make available government facilities, intellectual property, and expertise for collaborative interactions aimed at developing useful, marketable products that would benefit the public. The terms of a CRADA are usually brief and flexible so that each agreement can be negotiated and tailored to the needs and resources of the participating parties. There must be an intellectual contribution, which may take the form of materials, instrumentation, or expertise, from all parties to the agreement, but the federal government does not provide funding to nonfederal parties. However, a major benefit to an industrial collaborator is that it may obtain a first option for licensing of patents that result from the CRADA.

This type of agreement was recently used to establish a joint project between DOE and two companies—Celera and Compaq—to develop the next generation of software and computer hardware tools for computational biology (Washington Fax, January 29, 2001). Such bioinformatics tools

---

[27] See <http://materials.pnl.gov/CRADAs.htm>, and NIH Office of Technology Transfer, <http://ott.od.nih.gov/NewPages/crada-mn.html>.

are necessary to process data from large-scale projects such as the HGP, structural genomics, and proteomics. DOE will provide $10 million for work at Sandia National Laboratories. The exact financial contributions from the two firms have not been disclosed, but are also probably in the multimillion dollar range. Compaq and Sandia will work together on developing system hardware and software, while Celera and Sandia will collaborate on new visualization technologies for analyzing the massive quantities of experimental data generated by high-throughput instruments.

Nonprofit Funding of Large-Scale Biomedical Research

Nonprofit organizations, while making a small funding contribution in comparison with private industry and the government, have also played an important role in genomics research and could potentially contribute to other large-scale biology projects. Nonprofit[28] organizations come in a variety of different forms, including volunteer organizations, such as the American Cancer Society, that continually raise money to support research; endowed philanthropies, such as HHMI[29]; and even organizations set up by for-profit companies, such as the SNP Consortium. Examples of science-funding philanthropies are listed in Table 4-4. Profits generated by the bull stock market of the 1990s fueled unprecedented growth in philanthropic foundation assets and giving. In 1998, grant-making nonprofits spent more than $1 billion on science, but the recent downturn of the U.S. stock market has quelled that growth.

As noted earlier, philanthropies such as the Carnegie and Rockefeller Foundations played a leading role in funding and shaping basic science in the United States before World War II and by doing so even gave rise to new fields, such as molecular biology. Many organizations try to continue that tradition today by focusing on filling perceived gaps in federal funding and by defining highly specific targets for research (Cohen, 1999). In some ways, nonprofits have an advantage over government funding in their ability to change course quickly and to pursue nontraditional or high-risk projects. They often undertake peer review in a form much different from that of NIH, and some ignore the peer review process altogether. Many also have less-stringent reporting requirements with respect to progress and outcomes than does the federal government. While these characteristics may be considered risky at the very least, they certainly facilitate the fund-

---

[28]A nonprofit organization must spend 5 percent of its assets each year or face tax penalties.

[29]Because HHMI hires researchers as employees instead of awarding grants, it is in a different category and has to spend only 3.5 percent of its assets annually.

TABLE 4-4   Selected Science-Funding Philanthropies

Name	Founded	1999* Assets	1999* Science Expenses	Research Focus
Wellcome Trust	1936	$19.2B	$640M	Biomedical, no cancer
Bill and Melinda Gates Foundation	1994	$17.1B	$230M	Vaccines, reproductive medicine, public health
David and Lucile Packard Foundation	1964	$13.5B	$84.7M	Ocean sciences, computer science, math, natural science, engineering, interdisciplinary
Howard Hughes Medical Research Institute	1953	$12B	$427.7M	Biomedical
Pew Charitable Trusts	1948-79	$4.7B	$6.95M	Biomedical, neuroscience
Rockefeller Foundation	1913	$3.5B	$20M	Reproductive health, agriculture, vaccines, epidemiology, malaria
Andrew W. Mellon Foundation	1940-69	$3.5B	$3.1M	Contraception, repro- ductive biology, ecology
Kresge Foundation	1924	$2.1B	$4.6M	Scientific equipment
Carnegie Corporation	1911	$1.7B	$1M	Russian science
W. M. Keck Foundation	1954	$1.7B	$38.M1	Science, engineering, medical, astronomy
Donald Reynolds Foundation	1954	$1.4B	$35.2M over 5 years	Cardiovascular clinical research, geriatrics
Doris Duke Charitable Trust	1997	$1.4B	$13.8M	Physician-scientists, no animal research
Alfred P. Sloan Foundation	1934	$1.2B	$5.6M	Astronomy, molecular evolution, neurobiology, marine biology, compu- tational biology
Burroughs Wellcome Fund	1955	$669M	$35M	Biomedical
Edna McConnell Clark Foundation	1969	$640M	$898,000	Trachoma, onchocerciasis vaccine
Welch Foundation	1954	$362M	$23M	Chemistry, primarily in Texas
Carnegie Institution of Washington	1902	$527.1M	$31.4M	Astronomy, geophysics, plant biology, embryology
M. J. Murdock Charitable Trust	1975	$525M	$4M	Natural sciences, primarily in Pacific NW
James S. McDonnell Foundation	1950	$480M	$19M	Neuroscience, genetics, astronomy, complex systems
Arnold and Mabel Beckman Foundation	1977	$450M	NA	Chemistry, biochemistry, medicine

TABLE 4-4 *continued*

Name	Founded	1999* Assets	1999* Science Expenses	Research Focus
Whitaker Foundation	1975	$390M	$65.7M	Biomedical engineering
Charles A. Dana Foundation	1950	$311M	$10M	Neurosciences
Research Corporation	1912	$152.3M	$6.4M	Chemistry, physics, astronomy
Camille and Henry Dreyfus Foundation	1946	$125M	$3.4M	Chemistry
Ellison Medical Foundation	1998	N/A	100M over 5 years	Aging

*Many of these are estimates.
SOURCE: Cohen (1999).

ing of unconventional or controversial projects. With the exception of the largest organizations, such as HHMI, the Wellcome Trust,[30] and the Gates Foundation, however, single-handedly funding a large-scale initiative or providing long-term support beyond pilot projects may not be feasible. A joint venture is a possibility, but philanthropies often find it unpalatable to work together or with the federal government, fearing that they will dilute their own impact and identity (Cohen, 1999). Such was not the case, however, for the Wellcome Trust, which contributed heavily to several recent large-scale projects, including the internationally funded HGP. In most cases, investigators look to federal funding sources to continue a project that was launched successfully in a pilot or proof-of-principle stage using philanthropic sources. Such grant applications may then be viewed as less risky, but investigators may still encounter difficulties in obtaining NIH funds if the projects are very costly and the applications have not been solicited through a PA or RFA.

ISSUES ASSOCIATED WITH INTERNATIONAL COLLABORATIONS

The drive to achieve international standing and recognition in a particular field can promote competition and impede scientific cooperation. Nonetheless, the international collaborative approach for scientific re-

---

[30]The Wellcome Trust outspends the combined budgets of the United Kingdom's main government funders of biological research. Wellcome targets specific diseases, but avoids those that are relatively well funded (including cancer).

search has become commonplace for large-scale projects in such fields as high-energy physics, which require very large and expensive facilities. These collaborations may still be contentious because of competition among research groups or nations, but the end products of the research generally do not have direct commercial value. In the case of molecular biology and biomedical research, however, international competition is exacerbated by the fact that patents on new discoveries can be extremely lucrative. The lure of potential profits and market shares adds an additional level of complexity to negotiations for collaborative projects. These challenges are intensified by basic difficulties in organizing and managing projects undertaken on a global scale. Establishing uniform priorities and goals for the overall project and for each participant is highly problematic and is complicated by difficulties in communication across cultures, languages, and political environments.

Nonetheless, the scientific and engineering communities in the United States benefit from ideas and technologies developed around the world, and participating in international scientific and technical collaborations and exchanges may provide unique opportunities for addressing major problems or questions. Indeed, a 1995 NRC report recommends that the United States should pursue international cooperation to share costs, to tap into the world's best science and technology, and to meet national goals (National Research Council, 1995). The World Health Organization has led the way in creating structures to enable international cooperation for health R&D as a tool for economic and social development. According to the Global Forum for Health Research, the international activities budget for NIH increased steadily from 1991 to more than $200 million in 1998. There are international programs within the various NIH Institutes, but a breakdown of these activities was not available to the committee, and it is unclear how much of that funding went toward projects that would qualify as large-scale research as defined in this report.

SUMMARY

It is difficult, if not impossible, to quantify the total amount or proportion of biomedical research funding that is spent on large-scale research projects, primarily because of variation in definitions and reporting practices. As examples described here and in Chapter 3 clearly indicate, however, large-scale science projects are certainly being undertaken with funding from federal as well as nonfederal sources (the latter including industry and philanthropies and other nonprofits). The objectives and cultures of these different sources may vary considerably, yet partnerships among diverse funding sources could offer unique opportunities for undertaking large-scale endeavors if the challenges entailed can be overcome. In particular, public–private collaborations provide a way to share the costs and risks, as well as the benefits, of such efforts. International collaborations may present the greatest challenge of all, but also offer potentially unique opportunities. Some of the challenges involved, such as organization and management of projects and concerns about intellectual property, are covered in more detail in Chapters 5 and 7.

Federal funding for large-scale science projects continues to be controversial. Proposals for undertaking such projects often generate criticism and debate, both across and within fields. Although this debate on the relative value of such projects is crucial to their success, resolving these arguments is complicated by the fact that there is no consistent, established way to balance the allocation of funds across the various disciplines, or across big versus small projects. Over the course of the last century, however, scientists have come to expect federal funding for research, and those pursuing large-scale projects are no exception. Furthermore, former acting NIH director Ruth Kirschstein has noted that while the "bedrock" of the agency's research will continue to be individual investigator–initiated inquiry, the nature of scientific investigation is changing such that current research questions are more likely to require the efforts of multidisciplinary teams working with expensive instruments in specialized facilities (Haley, 2001). Similarly, current NIH director Elias Zerhouni has remarked that the model of the traditional NIH grant "will evolve into different shapes because multidisciplinary science requires collaborations." But he has also noted that "at the end of the day you also need [principal investigators] who themselves have an inherent understanding of [multiple] fields so they can ask the right questions" (Kaiser, 2002:1). According to Lake and Hood (2001), one of the outstanding challenges for contemporary biology is the integration of hypothesis-driven science with a new discovery approach to science—that is, defining all the elements of a biological system as a key information resource, and studying the entire system rather than asking questions about highly specific components.

The examples described in Chapter 3 indicate that there is flexibility within the NIH procedures that allows for some large-scale research endeavors. Within NIH, however, recent funding patterns suggest that perhaps only the Institutes with the largest budgets (e.g., NCI, NIGMS, and NHLBI) can independently handle the launch and support of a large-scale research project. Others may not have enough funds or flexibility in their budgets. For the smaller Institutes, undertaking such projects may require action and support on the part of the NIH director, or at least collaborative efforts among smaller and larger Institutes. NHGRI may be an exception to this generalization, since it was created specifically to undertake the large-scale HGP.

Some currently available funding mechanisms at NIH are amenable to large-scale projects and have already been used for such projects. Most of these efforts depended upon the solicitation of applications through PAs or RFAs that were issued for a specific topic of research. Unsolicited proposals for large-scale projects face what may be insurmountable obstacles in the form of grant size restrictions, traditional peer review expectations, and yearly fluctuations in the congressional allocations to NIH Institutes and Centers. Furthermore, using the R01 funding mechanism (the most common for unsolicited grants) for large-scale projects could lead to greater competition in the short term between scientists conducting large-scale and small-scale biomedical research because, absent a net increase in funding, each multimillion dollar grant would proportionally reduce the number of traditionally sized R01s awarded. As NIH approaches the completion of the budget doubling of recent years, there is already concern that the percentage of new applications funded will drop because of commitments made during the growth years (Korn et al., 2002; Jenkins, 2003b). At any given time, approximately 70 percent of the Institutes' funds are allocated for noncompeting renewals of awards made in previous years.

How are decisions to be made regarding the types of projects to be undertaken and the most pressing needs of the field? If NIH wishes to facilitate the process of funding large-scale projects that generate databases and other research tools, it may be helpful to change, or in some cases standardize, the decision-making procedures within the Institutes and Centers. For example, the traditional peer review process favor projects that are hypothesis driven. To date, in fact, none of the large projects funded by NCI have been reviewed through the CSR.[31] According to Craig Venter, the traditional dogmatic approach to peer review denies that biology is descriptive and impedes the progress of discovery (Lewis, 2001). While no one would deny the value of hypothesis-driven research, balancing the research portfolio with multiple approaches could enhance the progress of science overall. Changes in the peer review process could provide a first step in achieving that balance. A critical assessment and standardization of the procedures for issuing PAs and RFAs would also be useful for facilitating the funding of large-scale projects, since those mechanisms are currently the primary means of funding such projects. There is a need for a mechanism through which input from innovators in research can be routinely collected and incorporated into institutional decision-making processes as well.

A possible alternative to issuing PAs or RFAs for large-scale projects

---

[31] Personal communication, Richard Klausner, former NCI director.

aimed at particular topics would be to develop a special category, with specific review criteria and oversight requirements, for large-scale projects in general. Doing so would greatly speed the process for researchers with novel ideas while still maintaining a rigorous vetting process.

A third possibility would be to make greater use of Defense Advanced Research Projects Agency (DARPA)-type strategies for funding large-scale, technology-driven projects, as described in Chapter 3. NCI's Cancer Genome Anatomy Project and Unconventional Innovations Program could prove instructive in this regard. In any case, standardizing the methods for institutional oversight of such projects with regard to management structure and progress assessment over time would also improve the process, as is discussed in greater detail in Chapter 5.

A fourth potential mechanism to speed and facilitate the launch of large-scale projects would be to set up a loan program through NIH for the purpose of developing scientific infrastructure, such as new buildings or the purchase of expensive new technologies for research. Such a program would allow extramural institutions to react quickly to changing needs and opportunities in the field by securing funds from NIH early on, and then repaying the loan through traditional fundraising activities.

As noted in Chapter 3, several novel NIH programs have been launched in recent years in order to undertake large-scale research projects. These efforts depended on the institutional leadership at the time. Since many of those individuals have now left NIH, the future of such programs and the potential for launching other new programs is unclear. One way to reduce this variability is through long-term, Institute-wide strategic planning by the NIH director, as Elias Zerhouni is currently striving to do (Metheny, 2002; Kaiser, 2002). This planning process incorporates input from Institute and Center directors, as well as from leaders among intramural and extramural scientists in both academia and industry. Such an approach provides the best opportunity to ensure that NIH is responding effectively to changing needs in the field by funding innovative and useful projects in a timely fashion.

5

Organization and Management of Large-Scale Biomedical Research Projects

In the fields of biology and biomedical research, formal management of projects and staff traditionally has not been a major topic of concern, nor has it been widely studied. Training in management practices has been quite rare for Ph.D. candidates, and direct assessment of an investigator's managerial skills has played little or no role in promotion decisions or in the review of grant applications. The traditional structure of academic research laboratories, consisting of a single, independent principal investigator who oversees a small number of trainees (graduate students and postdoctoral fellows) and technicians, has been thought to present little need for hierarchical or formalized management methods. Furthermore, managerial oversight of investigator-initiated research by funding organizations has been minimal or nonexistent. With the advent of larger-scale projects that involve more scientists and larger budgets, however, effective management, both scientific and administrative, has become more important. This is especially true when multiple principal investigators and multiple institutions join forces to pursue a common mission or goal. In such collaborative efforts, it can be quite challenging to ensure that all the components of a project fit together and work effectively toward a collective goal. Project leaders must strive for a common vision and cultural integration among the various participants, who may include scientists and managers from different disciplines or different sectors, such as academia, industry, and government agencies.

Unfortunately, there is little information to guide the establishment of good managerial practices in such cases. This is due in part to the variability of research programs and goals, which makes it difficult to set uniform guidelines. In addition, the management of science, even in large-scale projects, has not been widely studied or assessed. Indeed, even in such fields as high-energy physics, in which large-scale, multi-institutional collaborations have been the norm for decades, the issue of research management has garnered little attention from scholars and remains a concern for scientists (National Research Council, 2001b). According to the American Institute of Physics (1992) "without a dedicated effort to understand [these complex] collaborations, policy makers and administrators will continue to have only hearsay and their own memories to guide their management. . . " (page 3).

The issue of research management is now coming to the fore because of increased demand by the government to account for the way federal funds are being used (see Chapter 4). The current Bush Administration is adamant about applying performance standards to assess the management and productivity of both large and small research endeavors. According to John Marburger, Director of the White House Office of Science and Technology Policy, performance measurement is "an inevitable as well as an essential aspect" of the relationship between the government and scientific research. In particular, he notes that "individuals dependent on large facilities bear the heavy responsibility of making judicious choices, ensuring prudent management and optimizing the quotient of discovery versus dollars" (Hafner, 2002: page 1).

EXAMPLES OF MANAGEMENT ASSESSMENT FOR LARGE-SCALE PROJECTS

Assessment of Federally Funded Laboratories

A recent study of federally funded U.S. research and development (R&D) laboratories examined their structure, management, and output through surveys and case studies, and revealed a great variety of organizational designs (Crow and Bozeman, 2001). Although a large portion of the laboratories examined were not performing biomedical research, there may be some applicable lessons to be learned from the study results. The authors of the study found that a proliferation of large research centers after the 1980s had resulted in new institutional and organizational designs. For example, there are now more collaborative research facilities and multi-sector centers, such as university–industry partnerships. In addition, there are more core user facilities and equipment- or process-driven centers. Technology development and technology transfer are also more common.

These newer types of research facilities and collaborations required a concomitant change in the approach to management. Before the emergence of research centers, most federally funded research was undertaken on a smaller scale by individual investigators conducting discipline-oriented projects. As a result, scientists who became center directors often lacked management experience, and some large-scale organizational needs suffered as a result. Furthermore, there appeared to be few mechanisms for diffusing managerial knowledge, and almost no incentive to do so. Rather, the authors of the study concluded that successful management approaches emerged from blind variation and selective retention (Crow and Bozeman, 2001). The study found that the partition of center management and scientific leadership (analogous to the chief scientist in industry) was quite effective. It also revealed that selecting research directions through a combination of traditional peer review and a nontraditional emphasis on building research capacity worked well.

With regard to funding, the authors concluded that the stability of funding is often more important than the actual amount of funding, as it provides a core for long-term planning and the development of support systems. Stable funding also facilitates "capacity evaluation" rather than "output evaluation." The distinction is important because government funding managers generally need to think in terms of projects and grants, but research managers often think in terms of resources and work activity. This divergence leads to a conundrum of trying to maintain the effectiveness of competitive peer review without stifling the productivity of research centers. Furthermore, determining a program's value within the environment of the Government Performance and Results Act (GPRA) is difficult when there are so many diverse contributions.

Evaluation of the National Science Foundation's Science and Technology Centers Program

Lessons may also be learned from an evaluation of the National Science Foundation's (NSF) Science and Technology Centers (STC) program. As described in Chapter 3, the STC program funds large-scale collaborative research that often is multidisciplinary and has broad, long-term goals. An extensive evaluation, including an assessment of organization and management, was conducted about 10 years after the program was initiated (National Academy of Public Administration, 1995, ABT Associates, 1996; National Research Council, 1996). A study panel appointed by the National Academies concluded that the success of the Centers is highly dependent on both their scientific and administrative management.[1] Because the Centers vary widely in their scope, objectives, research foci,

---

[1] The evaluation was based on site-visit reports, a survey of and interviews with the Center directors, and a previous report from the National Academy of Public Administration.

appropriate institutional linkages, and other characteristics, their management and organizational structures are also quite varied. However, effective oversight of the research programs present several common challenges for both Center directors and NSF program managers.

The National Academies panel found that a major challenge for the Center directors is to ensure that their Centers embody real collaboration and are not just groups of independent scientists working in a related area. A challenge for program leaders is to maintain focus over time. In a rapidly evolving field, for example, it can be difficult even for a successful Center that is meeting its initial goals to shift its focus in response to the field's natural evolution (e.g., from a basic to a more applied orientation or from one scientific emphasis to another). Moreover, any given Center may not be well constituted to make such large changes and remain successful. One of the greatest difficulties for NSF managers is ensuring that review and monitoring processes are effective. The panel concluded that site review by committees that include expert peers is very important, particularly in the first few years of a new program. The periodic site-review process was deemed very helpful in several cases when management problems occurred, as it assisted program leaders in identifying the problems and developing solutions (National Research Council, 1996).

SPECIAL CONSIDERATIONS FOR THE MANAGEMENT OF LARGE-SCALE BIOMEDICAL RESEARCH PROJECTS

Large-scale science clearly requires good management schemes and good managers. But what makes for a good manager, and what defines good management? Of course, there is no single response to this question, as the answer will vary depending on the project goal and the methods used to achieve that goal, both of which can be highly diverse. For example, the managerial needs of a large-scale project designed purely for the purpose of collecting data and creating a database to be used as a research resource may be quite different from those of a large-scale collaborative project addressing a complex research question. In general, project management entails four basic components:

- Setting goals and objectives
- Establishing a timeframe
- Planning, orchestrating, and coordinating activities to achieve the goals within that timeframe
- Evaluating progress toward the stated goals

However, the size, cost, complexity, and visibility of large-scale projects generate unique or heightened concerns and therefore demand greater stewardship and accountability than are characteristic of traditional small-scale projects.[2] Potential management problems tend to be proportional to the size of the project, and even apparently minor decisions could have major, precedent-setting implications for a large-scale project. As a result, planning and oversight become more labor- and time-intensive for the grant recipient as well as the funding agency, and thus the skills and commitment of both scientific and administrative managers for such projects are critical. For example, the funding agency must develop succinct and unambiguous terms for the award. Otherwise, it could be difficult to suspend or terminate a large-scale project once it has been launched, because of the visibility, politics, and sheer complexity of the undertaking. Agency staff must also define clearly the plans for monitoring and evaluating progress toward short-term milestones and long-term objectives, including potential actions to take when adequate progress is not being made, while still allowing enough flexibility to adapt to change as the work progresses. Oversight of many of the models described in Chapter 3 involves steering committees and advisory groups that include scientists who are well-respected peers in the field but are not directly involved in the projects. The extra responsibilities of the grant applicants include developing detailed, long-range plans to justify the large budget and the commitment of the funding agency. In fact, large-scale projects may require planning beyond a 5-year timeframe. Such long-range planning is extremely difficult in rapidly changing fields, and such timeframes are essentially unheard of even in the corporate world, where strategic planning is commonly undertaken (National Research Council, 1998).

When a large-scale project is carried out at multiple institutions or is funded by multiple sources, the complexities and difficulties associated with planning, coordination, monitoring, and assessment are exacerbated. Federal, industrial, academic, and nonprofit participants may each have their own priorities and ideas for how best to achieve their goals. Each funding source may also have different requirements for oversight or different stipulations for how to handle data release and intellectual property issues. Even when funding comes from multiple federal agencies, or perhaps even multiple Institutes within NIH, there can be disagreements over the roles and contributions of the various funders. This was certainly the case in the early efforts to launch the Human Genome Project, when the Department of Energy (DOE) and NIH were competing for funds and control of the project (reviewed by Davies, 2001; Cook-Deegan, 1994; Kevles and Hood, 1992). The leaders of a project must be able to commu-

---

[2] From STEP Administrative Strategies Forum: Big Science: Big Challenges, March 1, 2002, Bethesda, MD, National Institutes of Health.

nicate its vision in order to foster teamwork within the project and acceptance by the field as a whole.

Encouraging and maintaining open and effective communication among a project's various team members is also inherently challenging for large-scale, multi-institutional projects, especially when more than one discipline is involved. Participants must be able to speak the same language and need to trust each other enough to discuss ideas and work in progress. Several of the models described in Chapter 3 include regular meetings of the scientists working within collaborative projects, and this approach appears to be quite useful for facilitating good communication.[3] Such forums might be useful for collective decision making within large-scale projects as well. Advances in information technology (the Semantic Web, for example) may also facilitate communication within collaborative or multidisciplinary projects (Hendler, 2003).

Because the time commitment for principal investigators leading large-scale initiatives is likely to be much greater than is the case for more traditional projects (Mervis, 2002; Sulston and Ferry, 2002), it is often necessary to hire managers to oversee the day-to-day work of such a project. In academia, there appears to be a preference for managers with strong research credentials rather than strong management experience. However, there is no correlation between a person's abilities as a scientist and as a manager. Scientists are rarely trained to be managers, but it can also be argued that traditional business management training programs are not very applicable to the management of science because they are not adaptive enough (Austin, 2002). Conventional project management methods work best when the chances are good that a project will progress as expected. In contrast, science projects entail discovery and thus are more likely to require cyclical or iterative planning.

Effective scientist managers must have both technical and conceptual knowledge of the science involved in a project, in some cases in multiple disciplines, as well as good people skills, good judgment, and flexibility. The same is true of program managers within funding agencies. However, finding qualified individuals to take such positions can be difficult for a variety of reasons. Within academia, credit for a successful project may be given primarily to the principal investigator, even if the project manager has assumed significant responsibility. Furthermore, project managers, both in government agencies and in academia, do not necessarily have a sense of ownership of the data or other products of a project. Thus, taking on such a position could be a risky career

---

[3] Carol Dahl, former director of NCI's Unconventional Innovations Program, in a presentation to the National Cancer Policy Board, July 16, 2002.

move. Similarly, project management staff within federal agencies may not be viewed as scientific peers and may not be willing to assume the risks associated with managing a large-scale endeavor. Indeed, people with the right skills and qualifications for management positions are likely to find industry more appealing because of the career structure, incentives, and rewards for successful completion of a project[4] (see the section below for more detail). To address these issues, the National Laboratories use an alternative model encompassing dual career ladders that recognize and reward the achievements of managers who may not have the scientific credentials of top-tier researchers (Crow and Bozeman, 2001, see previous section). The National Laboratories also have a long history of managing large-scale projects for academic investigators and for rewarding scientists for their participation in team-oriented research.

THE INDUSTRY MODEL OF PROJECT MANAGEMENT: COMPARISON WITH ACADEMIA

The details of management approaches vary greatly depending on many factors, such as the environment in which the work is being done and the nature of the desired outcome. Historically, the approaches used most commonly in industry and academic settings are quite different.

In fact, the quintessential academic research project involves relatively little formal management beyond the individuals doing the work. The laboratory head or principal investigator is responsible for obtaining research funding through proposals that outline the objectives, methods, and expected timeframes of the project. He or she then oversees the work of one or a few graduate students, postdoctoral scientists, or technicians who perform the experiments. There is little or no oversight of the project by department or university officials or by officials of the funding agency. The overall work and productivity of the individual principal investigator are reviewed by university or department officials infrequently, such as when decisions regarding tenure or promotion are made. There is great variation across institutions in how the work of graduate students is evaluated; in the case of postdoctoral scientists, a recent survey indicates that most academic institutions do not require written performance evaluations or progress reviews (National Resource Council, 2000).

In contrast, most research undertaken in an industry setting involves

---

[4] Carol Dahl, former director of the NCI's Unconventional Innovations Program, in a presentation to the National Cancer Policy Board, July 16, 2002.

a team effort in which many investigators share similar levels of responsibility for bringing a single project to successful completion. There are many more layers of oversight and supervision, and everyone must work together toward a common goal. Progress is measured against written goals, a practice that promotes good planning and keeps everyone informed about what is expected of them. Generally, all members of the team are formally reviewed on an annual basis using a numerical ranking system that determines pay scales and advancement and is designed to elicit improvements from staff.[5] Such review may entail traditional top-down assessment of employees by their immediate supervisors. More recently companies have also been using another form of staff review known as "360 review" (see Box 5-1)—a method for assessing teamwork in which an employee's performance is evaluated by everyone in the circle that surrounds him or her, including peers, supervisors, and those who work for the employee (Edwards, 1996).

A significant obstacle to undertaking large-scale, collaborative projects within academia may be the inability of the current academic system to assess the work and productivity of individual team members and to reward those who make a significant contribution to a large-scale effort. For such work to be valued and respected, the criteria used for tenure, promotion, and hiring within academia would need to be changed or expanded to include a wider range of scientific achievements. A shift in emphasis away from measuring a scientist's success in obtaining traditional R01-type grants and toward an evaluation of research output and research capacity in the form of collaboration networks could facilitate such change. Perhaps the greatest obstacle to implementing this concept would be changing the mind-set of the reviewers who make decisions about promotions and tenure. However, there is at least some precedent for this approach in academia in the review of program grants (e.g., P01s), where the total research effort is expected to be greater than the sum of its individual components (see Box 4-7). Nonetheless, industry is still likely to have many more options at its disposal for recognizing and rewarding the work and contributions of team scientists through bonuses, pay increases, and opportunities for advancement within the company. Such career issues are discussed in greater detail in the following chapter.

---

[5] In some cases, a minimum or maximum number of employees must be assigned to the highest and lowest rankings to ensure that the ranking system is meaningful. For example, if a scale of 1–5 is used, with 1 being low and 5 being high, a group may be limited to no more than 15 percent of staff ranked as 5s while being expected to have a minimum of 5 percent of staff designated as 1s or 2s.

BOX 5-1   Hypothetical General Criteria That Could Be Used for Corporate Business "360 Performance Appraisal" Evaluation

Cognitive Reasoning Skills
- Problem solving
- Decision making
- Analyzing information
- Producing/following-through on ideas

Work Outcomes
- Time management
- Priority setting
- Meeting deadlines
- Setting/accomplishing objectives

Leadership Skills
- Motivates and supports team
- Develops team initiatives
- Fosters team progress
- Mentors junior team members

Personal Responsibility
- Personal initiatives
- Self-improvement
- Adaptable to change
- Knowledge development

Interpersonal Relationship Skills
- Teamwork
- Collaboration
- Communication

NOTE: Evaluation is based on employees' results and competencies.

SUMMARY

The capacity of large-scale biomedical research projects to make innovative and novel contributions to the field depends on their organizational structure and oversight. Because of their organizational complexity, cost, and visibility, large-scale projects have greater needs for management and oversight than is the case for more traditional biomedical research projects. Effective administrative management and scientific leadership are crucial for meeting expected milestones on schedule and within budget; thus the success of a large-scale project is greatly dependent upon the skills and knowledge of the scientists and administrators managing the project. Scientific managers must be well versed in the technical and conceptual aspects of the project, which may be multidisciplinary, and must also have exceptional organizational and communication skills to facilitate collaboration. However, it may be quite difficult to recruit scientists with the needed skill set into managerial positions because of the unusual status of such positions within the scientific career structure, and because scientists rarely undergo formal training in management. Furthermore, there is little information available on how to structure such management and oversight, and there are few precedents to follow in biomedical research.

To pursue large-scale endeavors in biomedical research effectively and efficiently, then, both universities and government agencies will need to develop incentives to encourage qualified scientists to take on the risks and responsibilities of managerial positions. Doing so could entail new approaches for assessing teamwork and management, as well as novel ways of recognizing and rewarding accomplishment in such positions. Both industry and the National Laboratories may serve as instructive models in achieving these goals, as they have a history of rewarding scientists for their participation in team-oriented research. Universities may need to define new faculty and staff categories that are consistent with this type of research, along with appropriate criteria for performance evaluation and promotion.

One attempt on the part of NIH to facilitate interdisciplinary teamwork is being undertaken by the Bioengineering Consortium (BECON), one of the few organizational units at NIH that crosses all Institutes and Centers. BECON is currently organizing a symposium called "Catalyzing Team Science," aimed at producing a set of guidelines for NIH on how to stimulate, facilitate, and reward collaborative efforts. The workshop will also include a discussion of academic institutions' assessment and reward procedures. It would also be expedient for NIH to formally assess the organization and management of its ongoing large-scale projects, as the National Science Foundation has done in the past. Such an exercise could perhaps lead to the formulation of guidelines for organizing and managing future large-scale projects more effectively or for assessing the management structure of proposed projects.

6

Training and Career Structures in Biomedical Research

R esearch at academic institutions traditionally has two primary objectives: to increase knowledge for the public good and to train the next generation of scientists. Thus, much of the research undertaken in academic laboratories is performed by "scientists in training," also known as graduate students, postdoctoral fellows, and clinical fellows. These trainees are expected to learn the essential skills of their field through direct experience—designing, conducting, and analyzing experiments or clinical studies under the supervision of an established scientist who serves as their mentor. Scientists who emerge from this training period and wish to follow the traditional academic career path of their mentors must obtain a tenure-track position and prove their ability to establish and maintain an independent research program, most often judged by their publication record and the amount of funding they obtain. The current system is well entrenched, and is designed primarily to produce new academic scientists to follow in their mentors' footsteps. As science changes, however, it may not always be the optimal approach for meeting the dual objectives of academic research. In fact, recent data indicate that only a minority of Ph.D. scientists establish a tenure-track career in academia (National Research Council, 1998b, 2000, 2001a). Many Ph.D. scientists work in non-tenure-track academic positions, in research positions in industry or government laboratories, or in other types of science-related jobs (see Figure 6-1 and 6-2). The recent emergence of large-scale projects in the biomedical sciences, in particular, could present significant challenges in meeting the needs of trainees and junior scientists, as the tradi-

A. One to three years since doctorate

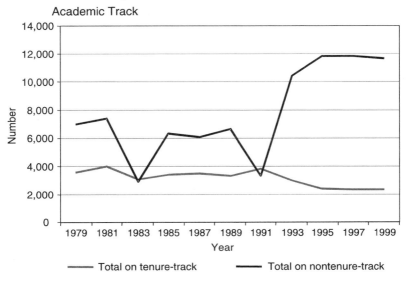

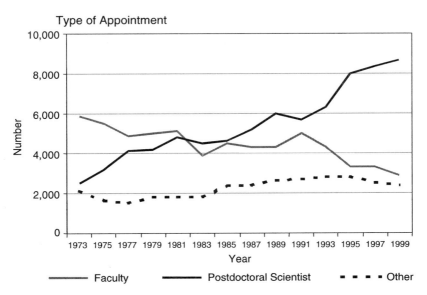

FIGURE 6-1   Number of recent science and engineering Ph.D.s employed in academia by type of appointment and academic track, 1973–1999. A: One to three years since doctorate. B: Four to seven years since doctorate.
SOURCE: National Science Foundation, 2002, Appendix Table 5-27.

B. Four to seven years since doctorate

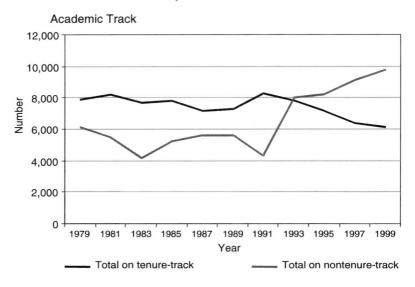

Academic Track

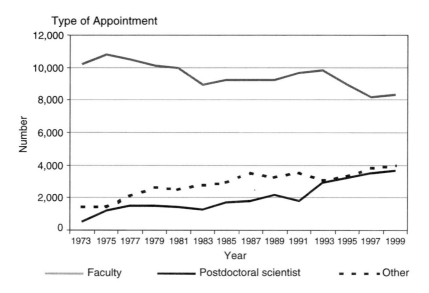

Type of Appointment

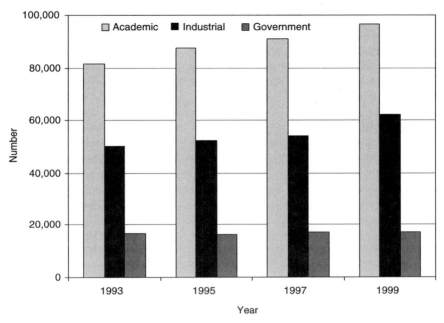

FIGURE 6-2   Life science Ph.D.s by employment sector.
SOURCE: National Science Foundation, 2002, Appendix Table 3-18.

tional structure of training and career paths in academic research may be at odds with efficient and effective endeavors in large-scale science.

The effects on the career trajectories of biomedical scientists of working within large-scale projects have not been studied, but by examining career issues more broadly in the field, it may be possible to identify potential obstacles faced by such scientists. This chapter provides an overview of the current system and the challenges it presents to scientists in general and to biomedical scientists in particular.

THE TRADITIONAL ACADEMIC TRAINING AND CAREER STRUCTURE IN BIOMEDICAL SCIENCE

The hierarchy of academic degrees dates back to the universities of thirteenth-century Europe, which had faculties organized into guilds (see Box 6-1). Degrees[1] were in effect professional certifications that faculty members had attained the guild status of a "master." The traditional aca-

---

[1] There was originally only one degree in European higher education, with the equivalent titles of either master or doctor.

BOX 6-1   The Medieval European Guild System

The European guild system, which flourished in Europe between the eleventh and sixteenth centuries, had two major periods of development. The first culminated in the merchant guilds, which were associations formed in nearly all towns for the purpose of managing and controlling trading and commerce. Such guilds were associations of all or most of the merchants dealing in various categories of goods in a particular town. The objective of the guild was to enable the merchants to maintain a monopoly in, and efficient organization of, all the merchandising in a given community. As industry developed in scope and complexity, it became increasingly difficult for these merchant guilds to retain their monopolies, so a new system of individual craft guilds gradually arose to supersede the old system of merchant guilds. Craft guilds were occupational associations that usually comprised all the artisans and craftsmen in a particular branch of industry. For example, whereas the merchant guild had organized the leather business as a whole, craft guilds broke it up into specialties, so that tanners, saddlemakers, harnessmakers, shoemakers, bootmakers, and so on each had their own guild. There was a struggle between the new guild system and the old, but the old at last gave way and ceased to exist in the fifteenth century.

The primary purpose of the craft guild was to establish a complete system of industrial control over all who were pursuing a given craft. The guild set and maintained standards for the quality of goods and the integrity of trading practices in that industry. The guild membership was divided into a hierarchy with three levels: masters, journeymen, and apprentices. Apprenticeship was an indentured method for training youths in a vocation. Upon completion of the indentured training, the apprentice graduated into the ranks of the journeymen. Passing to the higher grade was based on proof of skill, such as a "masterpiece" or an examination. A journeyman often hired himself out to a master for 2 or 3 years for wages and then, with a little money of his own, set up in his own shop, hired journeymen, indentured apprentices, and became a master.

Eventually the masters, being the wealthy class, tended to assume more and more power and to adopt legislation in their own interests. As the number of journeymen increased and a permanently wage-earning class developed, the journeymen began to form guilds of their own, often in spite of the authorities. This conflict between masters and journeymen frequently erupted into fierce battles and bloodshed.

The medieval craft guilds slowly declined during the Renaissance and Reformation periods. The guilds broke down as the pace of technological innovation spread, and new opportunities for trade disrupted their hold over a particular industry. Masters tended to become foremen or entrepreneurs, while journeymen and apprentices became paid laborers.

SOURCE: Encyclopedia Britannica, 2003; Haywood, 1923.

demic training experience in the United States can also be likened in some ways to the medieval European apprentice model of craft guilds, in which a master craftsman agreed to instruct a young person in exchange for shelter, food, clothing, and medical care. The apprentice would bind himself to work for the master for a given time. After the agreed-upon time period he would become a journeyman, working for a master for wages, or set up as a master himself. Similarly, a student interested in pursuing an advanced degree in the sciences most often enters as an "apprentice" or graduate student in an academic research laboratory and in a sense "binds" his or her training to one specific scientific mentor or "master." In return, the graduate student receives a stipend to cover basic living expenses and is offered intense training in the scientific discipline of the mentor. This training, which lasts a median of 7–8 years (National Research Council, 1998b), ideally integrates a broad array of professional activities, such as conducting research, writing articles and grants, and teaching. Compared with the medieval guilds that supervised the relation of master and apprentice and monitored the number of apprentices in a given guild, however, current arrangements between graduate students and their mentors in the life sciences are much less monitored or regulated.

Upon completion of graduate training, the next step on the traditional academic career track in the life sciences is most commonly a postdoctoral position—similar to that of a "journeyman"—in which scholars work on a full-time but temporary basis to gain additional research experience in preparation for a professional research career. The roots of postdoctoral training in the United States date back more than a century to the 1870s, when high-level apprenticeships became part of new research institutions modeled after European examples. The postdoctoral fellowship is essentially a hybrid of the German privatdocent and the English fellowship, in which scientists acquire skills, prove themselves as independent scientists, and seek faculty openings (Hackett, 1987). The Johns Hopkins University adopted the apprenticeship model shortly after its founding in 1876, and in the 1920s the Rockefeller Foundation established formal postdoctoral fellowships in physical science, recognizing that physics had become too complex to learn within the time limits of traditional programs.

After a postdoctoral fellowship, the next step in a customary academic career path is securing a tenure-track faculty position (National Science Foundation, 2002). Traditionally, tenure has guaranteed the permanence of a faculty position awarded upon successful completion of a probationary period, usually 7 years. Tenure was designed to enforce academic freedom and to make an academic career more attractive by providing job security. In practice, however, tenure in the biomedical sciences provides minimal job security because it does not come with a guarantee of laboratory space or money for research.

The tenure process is usually quite rigorous and can sometimes span the entire career of a faculty member. The usual professorial series, which forms the core of most academic faculty, consists of three ranks: assistant professor, associate professor, and full professor. Each rank is divided into steps of a review process. Professorial advancement up the ladder is not guaranteed and is commonly based on a multilevel merit review system that varies from one institution to another. Faculty members are usually evaluated on four main criteria: research and creative work, professional competence and activity, teaching, and university and public service. In the life sciences, assessment of the first two criteria is most critical, and generally entails a review of the professor's publication record and level of funding. The multilevel review system most often involves contributions from the individual, the department, the dean, academic senate committees, and the chancellor or vice chancellor. This multilevel procedure is intended to ensure that colleagues and administrators evaluate the professional achievements of the individual in a balanced way and in accordance with clearly defined procedures.

An example of a tenure review process, used by the University of California system, is described in Box 6-2. In this case, new assistant professors are appointed initially to a 2-year contract and have a maximum of 8 years to demonstrate excellence as scholars and earn tenure. At 2-year intervals during this probationary period, candidates are evaluated and informed of their strengths and weaknesses. A midcareer appraisal, generally during the fourth year, is the major performance evaluation before the tenure review. The tenure review, which generally occurs in the sixth or seventh year, leads to the chancellor's final decision on whether to grant tenure. Both the midcareer appraisal and the tenure review include the solicitation of evaluations from experts outside the university.

While the granting of tenure may be the most important decision affecting a faculty member's career, the post-tenure merit-based review system has recently entered the academic tenure structure at many institutions and has become a hotly debated national issue, especially as it pertains to the philosophy of academic freedom. At several institutions, it is common for an associate professor to be reviewed every 2 years, and after approximately 6 years to undergo a full review, similar in complexity to the tenure review, for promotion to full professor. The intent of this continuing review process is to maintain the excellence of the faculty and to reward faculty members on the basis of merit (Box 6-2).

BOX 6-2   An Example of Tenure Review: The University of California

Preparation of the Personnel File
1. Department chair advises the candidate on the review process.
2. The candidate compiles for the department a review file that includes:
   - The candidate's research and/or publications to date.
   - A bio-bibliography documenting the candidate's university service and public service.
   - Information on teaching, courses taught, independent study, and supervision of graduate students.

Review by the Department
1. The department chair adds evaluations from students to the candidate's file.
2. The department chair solicits appraisals of the candidate from external reviewers, and the anonymous written responses are placed in the file.
3. The candidate may inspect all documents in the file that are not confidential. Upon request, the department chair will provide a redacted copy of confidential academic review records to the candidate.
4. The candidate may submit a written response to the materials in the file.
5. The department reviews the candidate's file and votes to recommend for or against tenure for the candidate.
6. The department chair may add an independent recommendation of his or her own.
7. The department chair informs the candidate of the department's recommendation and the substance of the departmental evaluations for each of the criteria (teaching, research, professional activity, and university and public service).
8. The candidate may make a written comment on the department's recommendation.

Review Beyond the Department
1. The candidate's review file, with the department's recommendation, is submitted to the dean for review.
2. The dean's recommendation is added to the file along with that of the department, and the file is forwarded to the appropriate academic senate committee (the committee on academic personnel or equivalent committee).
3. The committee on academic personnel nominates an ad hoc committee of experts in the candidate's discipline; the chancellor or vice chancellor formally appoints this ad hoc committee to review the candidate's file.
4. After reviewing the ad hoc committee's analysis and recommendation, the committee on academic personnel adds its own recommendation to the file along with those of the department and dean, and forwards the file to the chancellor or his/her designee to review.
5. The chancellor or designee reviews the recommendations from previous reviewers and makes the decision to grant or deny tenure to the candidate. If there is not consensus, the deciding officer and the committee on academic personnel consult.

This multilevel review process with input from multiple faculty groups (the department, the committee on academic personnel, and the ad hoc committee) and from multiple administrators (the department chair, the dean, and the chancellor or designee), combined with evaluations of reviewers from outside the university, is an element of the system of shared governance that is designed to select and promote an outstanding faculty.

SOURCE: University of California, 1997.

OVERVIEW OF TRENDS IN THE BIOSCIENCE WORKFORCE

Ph.D. Scientists

Over the last several decades, dramatic shifts have occurred in the U.S. scientific workforce. The number of Ph.D.'s awarded annually in the life sciences has more than tripled since the 1960s (National Research Council, 1998b; see Figure 6-3). In fact, almost all of the growth in Ph.D. production in the United States in the last several decades has been in the biomedical fields. In the last 15 years, an increasing percentage of these degrees have been awarded to citizens of other nations, more than half of whom choose to remain in this country (National Research Council, 1998b; National Science Foundation, 2000; see Figure 6-4). During this same period, tenure-track faculty positions have declined sharply, and the number of full-time non-faculty or non-tenure-track positions has increased (National Science Foundation, 2000; Hackett, 1987). The shift to such positions could potentially have a negative impact on the field as a whole in a variety of ways, including reduced autonomy and security for early-career scientists (see Box 6-3). Two net results of these combined changes are an increase in the length of postdoctoral training and a marked reduction in the opportunity for Ph.D. scientists to obtain a tenure-track faculty position. Ph.D. scientists in research universities are now more likely to be in non-tenure-track positions than to have tenure-track faculty appointments (National Science Foundation, 2002; see Figure 6-1). In the life sciences, which account for about two-thirds of all postdoctoral scientists in the United States, a postdoctoral appointment can last 3 to 5 years or

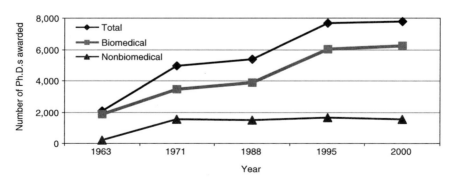

FIGURE 6-3 Number of U.S. life science Ph.D.s awarded annually, by broad field, 1963–2000.
SOURCE: National Research Council, 1998; National Science Foundation, 2002.

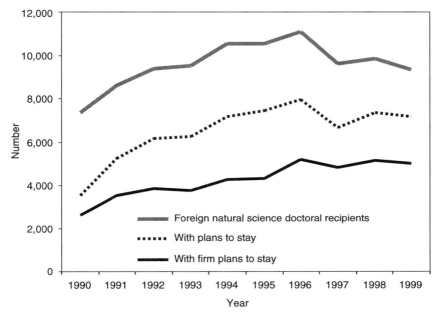

FIGURE 6-4   Foreign doctoral recipients in natural science with plans to stay in the United States, 1990–1999.
SOURCE: National Science Foundation, 2002, Appendix Table 2-32.

more, and it is not unusual for an individual to assume multiple consecutive postdoctoral positions. Concomitantly, the average age of scientists receiving NIH grant support has increased dramatically. The percentage of grants going to scientists under age 35 has declined steadily —from 23 percent in 1980 to 4 percent in 2001—while the percentage going to scientists aged 46 and older has grown sharply—from about 20 percent to about 60 percent (Goldman and Marshall, 2002).

Although other career options besides academic tenure-track positions exist for Ph.D. scientists (e.g., in industry, funding agencies, patent law, science writing), a recent survey indicates that the majority of doctoral students enter their graduate program with an interest in a faculty career (Golde and Dore, 2001). Thus there is intense competition for the academic positions available, similar to that seen in a tournament (Freeman et al., 2001). Like an Olympic sporting event, a tournament amplifies small differences in effort, ability, or productivity into large differences in recognition and reward, intensifying the competition and creating a disproportionate incentive to win (Lazear and Rosen, 1981). In the case of biomedical research, an independent career in academia might represent

---

**BOX 6-3   Excerpt from "The Plight of Academic Marginals"
by E. J. Hackett
(*The Scientist*, July 27, 1987)**

Major universities employ many Ph.D.s in academically marginal positions, neither postdocs nor full-fledged faculty. . . .Marginal positions can be regarded as an extension of the scientific apprenticeship system, which includes graduate education and postdoc fellows. But the marginal jobs fall far short of an ideal scientific apprenticeship. For example, such positions may not provide the freedom and resources necessary to become properly apprenticed as a scientist. The constraints, measured in terms of both budget and autonomy, are often so great that the appropriate skills are not acquired. Similarly, some marginals have suggested that the socialization is not adequate—that the right rules are not taught—thus, failing at another function of the apprenticeship. Moreover, these positions may not lead to secure employment.

More serious questions arise from the traditional use of apprenticeships to restrict the flow and shape the characteristics of new workers entering a craft. In science the hiring of people into marginal positions (and their dismissal from them) may be less formal than hiring into faculty slots, and carry fewer formal protections of individuals' rights. And whatever the formal guidelines for the treatment of such people on the job, it is very likely that informal norms and practices have substantial power.

These marginal positions are a variant of the postdoctoral fellowship. Marginal positions are a product of federal research support and, as changes in support are used as an instrument of science policy, these scientists' careers are redirected, perhaps in unintended and undesirable ways. In effect, we may be restructuring the academic career in a self-defeating fashion, removing some autonomy and many of the rewards from the early career while building in a career change at the wrong time. Or we may be restructuring academia, adding a new layer of professional whose rights and status are now under negotiation. A sensible science policy requires a better understanding of such marginal positions and their role in U.S. science and education.

---

the "prize." In an ideal setting, tournament job markets can be socially efficient, inducing high productivity from all participants. Given the current career structure of biomedical science, however, the tournament market incentives involved tend to benefit senior investigators at the expense of new entrants (Freeman et al., 2001).

Postdoctoral scientists with foreign citizenship may be especially vulnerable within this system. The number of foreign nationals taking postdoctoral positions in the United States has quadrupled since the mid-1970s (National Research Council, 1998b, 2001a). In recent years, half of all postdoctoral scientists in academia and in NIH intramural laboratories have been foreign citizens (National Research Council, 1998, 2000). The status of these postdoctoral scientists is determined to a large extent by their visa. The most common visa options[2]—the "J" student visa and the "H" professional visa—both have substantial drawbacks when applied to postdoctoral scientists (National Research Council, 2000). For example, NIH training grants cannot support foreigners on student visas. In addition, foreign nationals on a J visa commonly depend on their advisors for visa extensions or conversion to a green card, creating the potential for abuse. To complicate matters, when mentoring problems arise, foreign postdoctoral scientists may be restricted from changing advisers.

Some data indicate that foreign nationals in the United States can compete well for positions beyond the postdoctoral level. Data collected by the Association of American Medical Colleges indicate that nearly one-third of new hires of Ph.D.s and M.D.s in basic science departments in the late 1980s and in the 1990s were foreign nationals (National Research Council, 1998b). However, making the transition from a postdoctoral position to more permanent employment can be difficult because of visa issues. For example, the H work visa, which has a time limit of 6 years, requires that a petition be filed with the Immigration and Naturalization Service by a company or organization in the United States, and the application is filed for positions rather than for particular individuals.

The supply of Ph.D.s in the life sciences in the United States is inevitably linked to the demand for work in laboratories because of the interconnectedness of training and work in the field (Freeman et al., 2001). Postdoctoral scholars and graduate students make economical and effective workers in the laboratory because they are motivated by the hope of achieving an independent research career and making important contributions, rather than by monetary incentives. Thus the performance of research in the United States has relied more and more on Ph.D. scientists in training or non–tenure-track positions. As a whole, this portion of the workforce has become indispensable to the scientific enterprise, performing a substantial portion of the nation's research. In many laboratories, these "junior" scientists help write grant proposals and papers; present the laboratory's research results at professional society meetings; and also educate, train, and supervise other members of the laboratory (National Research Council, 1998b, 2000). Indeed, a 1999 survey of research articles published in *Science* found that 43 percent of the first authors were in postdoctoral positions (Vogel, 1999).

Shifts in the Ph.D. workforce have been driven largely by increased funding for biomedical science, which has led to more grants that include money to pay for the stipends of trainee research assistants working on the funded project. Over the last 25 years, the number of graduate stu-

---

[2] See <http://travel.state.gov/nonimmigrantvisas.html>.

TABLE 6-1   Number and Percentage of Graduate Students of Various
Kinds and Sources of Support, 1975 and 1995

	1975		1995	
	No.	% of group	No.	% of group
Federal support				
Research assistant	4,653	41.7	11,963	66.5
Trainee/fellow	5,944	53.6	5,391	30
Teaching assistant	118	1.1	155	0.9
Other	404	3.6	471	2.6
Total federal	**11,119**	**100.0**	**17,980**	**100.0**
Institutional support				
Research assistant	3,876	25.3	8,489	38.2
Trainee/fellow	2,040	13.3	4,017	18.1
Teaching assistant	8,495	55.5	8,589	38.6
Other	901	5.9	1,136	5.1
Total institutional	**15,312**	**100.0**	**22,231**	**100.0**
Other				
Self-supported	9,359	71.8	6,396	55.5
Private and foreign	3,676	28.2	5,124	44.5
Total other	**13,035**	**100.0**	**11,520**	**100.0**
Grand Total	**39,466**	**100.0**	**51,731**	**100.0**

SOURCE: National Research Council, 1998:26.

dents supported as research assistants through federal or institutional
funding awarded to principal investigators has increased greatly, while
the number of students supported directly by federal training grants or
fellowships has decreased (National Research Council, 1998b; see Table
6-1). The number of postdoctoral positions supported on principal investigator grants is even greater (National Science Foundation, 2002), reflecting the relatively heavy use of postdoctoral scientists in university-based
biomedical research, as well as the growth of independent research institutes, which hire postdoctoral scientists but do not train graduate students. The vast majority of postdoctoral scientists work in universities
(see Figure 6-5) as research associates on principal investigator grants, but
the exact number of grant-supported postdoctoral positions is unclear
because different institutions use different titles to describe them. Furthermore, major funding agencies (e.g., the National Science Foundation
[NSF] and NIH) do not have a mechanism for counting or tracking postdoctoral scientists (National Research Council, 2000).

NIH does make an effort to track graduate students and postdoctoral
scientists supported by training grants and fellowships (the National Re-

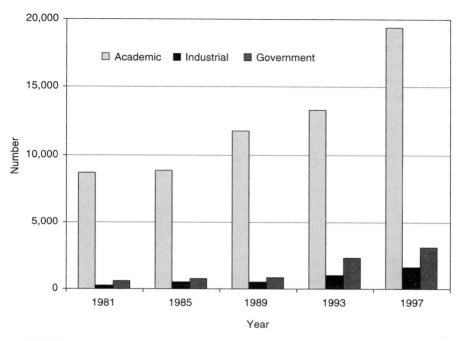

FIGURE 6-5   Number of postdoctoral appointments across employment sectors, 1981–1997.
SOURCE: National Research Council, 2001, Table B-2.

search Service Awards, or NRSA), but it currently does not track trainees supported by grants to principal investigators. NIH is experimenting with an electronic data system that could potentially track all trainees, but that tool is not likely to be widely used in the near future (see Box 6-4). And even in the case of NRSA fellows, NIH currently does not distinguish among different scientific specialties or characterize the recipients by other variables that could indicate the size and scope of their projects. Most universities do not track the career progression of their Ph.D. graduates or postdoctoral scientists, either[3] (Freeman et al., 2001). As a result, little information is available for assessing the effects of different work environments or projects on the career trajectories of junior scientists.

There is also a paucity of data available on scientists who work in

---

[3] This is in contrast to most professional schools (e.g., law, business, medicine) associated with major universities, which track the careers of their graduates and make the resulting information available to the public.

BOX 6-4   Tracking Trainees with the NIH X-Train System

NIH is setting up an electronic data system called X-Train that will be used to track National Research Service Award (NRSA) trainees. Graduate students and postdoctoral fellows with NRSA funding will fill out an electronic professional profile (PPF) with demographic and professional information, such as degree, position title, and publications. This electronic professional profile, similar to the biosketch required on all grant applications, will be supplemented by the principal investigator who will provide the training appointment. X-Train is currently in use on a trial basis at about 13 institutions, and should be completed and launched in the spring of 2003.

NIH is also working on a second version of X-Train that could be used to track all trainees (students and postdoctoral fellows) associated with principal investigator grants. Trainees will fill out the electronic PPF, which will be supplemented by the principal investigator on the grant application. This procedure will start on a voluntary basis; compliance will be assessed by NIH, which will determine whether the procedure should become mandatory. NIH should be able to track the progress of trainees from student to postdoctoral fellow to principal investigator using the resultant database, as long as the individual in the PPF remains in the NIH system. However, a definitive date for implementation of this second version of X-Train has not been set.

SOURCE: Walter Schaffer, NIH Office of Fellowships and Grants. Presentation to the IOM National Cancer Policy Board, October 7, 2002.

---

other non–tenure-track positions, although they make up a substantial fraction of the scientific workforce at many universities, especially medical schools (Barinaga, 2000). Like postdoctoral positions, these positions come with titles ranging from researcher or research associate to adjunct or in-residence professor. What they have in common is that grants rather than their institutions pay the salaries of these individuals, and they have little or no long-term job security. The majority of non–tenure-track scientists work within collaborative groups, so most positions are under the support and supervision of a tenured faculty member. One advantage of such positions may be the opportunity to work within a well-funded premier research team doing cutting-edge science. On the other hand, these scientists may be quite limited in their ability to establish an independent reputation for the work they perform or to reap the rewards of scientific accomplishment. Some positions do come with independent investigator status, but even those who have established successful independent research programs from such positions often report a feeling of "second-class citizenship" compared with tenured faculty in their institutions (Barinaga, 2000).

M.D. Scientists

There are no comprehensive sources of data for examining the factors influencing the education and career outcomes of physician scientists. However, several recent studies have examined data from a variety of sources and reached similar conclusions—that the number of physician scientists is not keeping pace with the recent expansion of biomedical research, leading to a scarcity of physicians trained to undertake clinical research (Zemlo et al., 2000; Heinig et al., 1999; Institute of Medicine, 1994, 2000; Nathan, 1997). Although the number of M.D.s in clinical departments of medical schools did increase between 1980 and 1994, the fraction of NIH-funded researchers in clinical departments who are physician scientists has declined (Zemlo et al., 2000). Moreover, although the number of NIH grants going to M.D. applicants increased by 32 percent between 1970 and 2001, the fraction of NIH research project awards to physician scientists declined steadily until the mid-1980s and remained level since then[4] (Heinig et al., 1999), despite the fact that M.D.s are as successful as Ph.D.s in securing NIH research grants (see Figure 6-6).[5] Perhaps more telling are indications that the number of first-time physician applicants for NIH funding has declined sharply in recent years, and that these applicants are far less likely than Ph.D. applicants to modify and resubmit their proposals (Nathan, 1997).

As in the case of the increasing number of Ph.D. life scientists, these opposite, downward trends in the number of physician scientists are associated with financial issues, but of a different sort. As teaching and research hospitals grapple with the new realities of cost containment and managed care policies, they require more patient care time from their medical faculty, leaving less time for research. These expectations, combined with the relatively long training period for a research career and the large debts upon completion of professional training, have apparently discouraged many new M.D.s from following a research career path, which is likely to provide a lower salary than a clinical career path (Zemlo et al., 2000; Heinig et al., 1999; Institute of Medicine, 1994, 2000; Nathan, 1997).

---

[4] The number of grants going to M.D. applicants increased from 1,202 to 2,839 between 1970 and 2001. The number of grants awarded to Ph.D. applicants increased by 68 percent during the same time period, from 1,960 to 6,137 (see <http://grants2.nih.gov/grants/award/trends/mdsphds7001.htm>).

[5] Based on NIH-wide averages of success rates for competing research project grants. Paylines at NIH vary greatly both across and within Institutes and Centers, depending on the review section and type of grant. For example, in fiscal year 2002, the overall success rate for NCI grant applicants was 29 percent, but R01s were funded to the 22nd percentile, while P01s were funded to the 40th percentile.

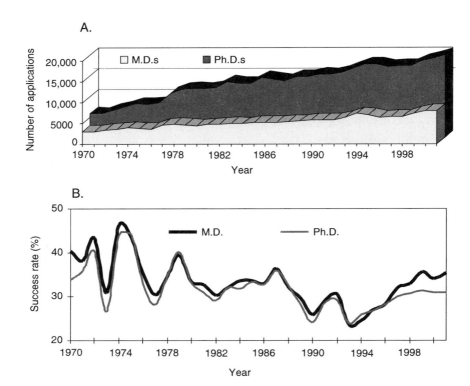

FIGURE 6-6   NIH competing research project applications by degree. A: number of applications. B: Success rate (NIH-wide averages). NOTE: M.D. category contains M.D./Ph.D.s.
SOURCE: <http://grants.nih.gov/grants/award/trends/mdsphds/001.html>.

Several other challenges have been suggested as obstacles to successful careers in clinical research in particular. These include the complexity of working with human subjects; the long timeframe involved in many studies; and the requirement for the involvement of multiple investigators, which leads to difficulties in assigning credit for papers with multiple authors (Shine, 1998). At the University of California-San Francisco (UCSF), focus groups reported that, with regard to promotions, serving as an essential collaborator on a project with other principal investigators was valued less than work done under an independent NIH R01 grant. They also noted that this difficulty was exacerbated by departmental policies that discouraged members from submitting grant proposals through organized research units or functioning as coinvestigators on grants to members of other departments (Task Force on the Future of Clinician Scientists at UCSF, 2000). A lack of adequate mentoring has also been identified as a possible cause for the decline of clinical scientists (Zemlo et al., 2000; Task Force on the Future of Clinician Scientists at UCSF, 2000).

POTENTIAL IMPACT OF LARGE-SCALE RESEARCH ON BIOMEDICAL TRAINING AND CAREER STRUCTURES

Because large-scale projects can vary greatly in their objectives and methods, it is not possible to generalize the career- or training-related obstacles to all cases. Each project may involve unique considerations. Noted here are a variety of potential issues that may arise within large-scale projects in biomedical research.

As discussed in the previous chapter, large-scale projects require different management structures and oversight as compared with the more traditional small-scale projects. As a result, principal investigators who receive funding to undertake a large-scale project often need to hire scientific managers for the project. It can be difficult to recruit such people, as they must be well versed in the science and technology of the project and also have managerial skills, which are generally not taught in life science training programs. Furthermore, because of the high costs and high profile of large-scale projects, the expectations for such scientist managers are very high, yet adequate incentives and compensation may be lacking, both professionally and financially. Because these scientists are funded through the grant to the principal investigator of the project, they are not likely to be on the tenure-track, so they have relatively little job stability if funding for the project is cut. If they are successful in overseeing the project to completion, most of the credit is likely to go to the principal investigator, and there may be little opportunity for promotion or other types of compensation that one finds in industry—where salaries for such managers are also considerably higher. Even if the project managers are on tenure-track, participation in large collaborations may not be valued as highly by review committees as more traditional, independent work. The same is true for junior faculty (M.D.s or Ph.D.s who are on tenure-track but not yet tenured) who join a project as collaborating investigators.

Graduate students and postdoctoral scientists who work on large-scale endeavors could be at risk because such projects may have a timeframe that does not fit readily with normal training programs. They may invest large amounts of time and effort, only to emerge with little to show for that investment with respect to a publication record or a scientific reputation that would help them land a position on the next rung of the career ladder. Even if publications do result from the work, the papers often include many collaborative authors, so the specific contributions of trainees may be difficult to ascertain. In addition, generating pools of data for a large-scale project may be very labor-intensive and can entail a great deal of extremely repetitive work. Although laboratory research in general can often be repetitive and tedious in day-to-day practice, the scale and scope of very large projects can amplify this characteristic—for example, by focusing primarily on a single method. As a result, trainees may not obtain the needed variety of experience in their training when working within such projects.

The Human Genome Project provides a clear example of many of these issues. As noted in Chapter 3, the project was initially organized in the traditional fashion, with principal investigators being funded to undertake small pieces of the overall project. Much of the work was performed by graduate students and postdoctoral scientists, who were expected to learn and carry out all the necessary procedures for mapping and sequencing a particular region of the genome. But progress on the project was slower than expected, so there was considerable incentive to streamline the process to meet projected deadlines, particularly after Celera provided competition for the public project (see Chapter 3; Sulston and Ferry, 2002). As a result, funding was redirected toward a few major centers that were reorganized using an industrial model. Many non-Ph.D. technicians were hired to perform the repetitive work within core groups based on specific methods, and a small number of Ph.D. scientists were hired as scientific managers. Graduate students and postdoctoral scientists were largely removed from the data-gathering aspects of the project.[6] When the draft sequence of the public project was published in *Nature*, the paper included more than 250 names (Lander et al., 2001).[7] Whether all of these authors met the usual academic standards for authorship is not known, but even if only a fraction of them did, the author list would still be considerably longer than is typical of a paper in the biosciences.

The fate of the graduate students and postdoctoral scientists who worked on the Human Genome Project in the early years of the project is unknown because they have not been tracked. One might perhaps predict that such individuals would have fared better than the average life scientist, since the field of genomics is very new and expanded rapidly in conjunction with the project. In fact, individuals with training in bioinformatics were in short supply and highly sought after as the field of genomics expanded (Stephan and Black, 2001). A review of available positions in genomics, proteomics, structural biology, and bioinformatics advertised in two randomly chosen issues of *Science* magazine in 2001

---

[6] Trainees with an interest in bioinformatics were still involved in data analysis.

[7] The paper published by the Celera team also included more than 250 authors.

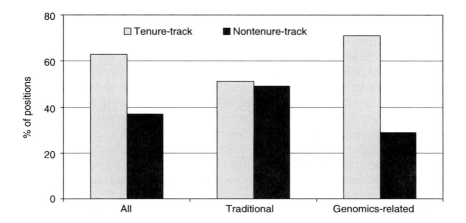

FIGURE 6-7   Percent of tenure and nontenure positions requiring a Ph.D. advertised in two randomly chosen volumes of *Science* (Vol. 292 [5523], Vol. 293 [5537]). NOTE: Traditional positions include listings for cell biology, molecular biology, and biochemistry. Genomics-related positions include genomics, proteomics, bioinformatics, and structural biology listings.

actually showed a high percentage of tenure-track positions (see Figure 6-7) compared with the more traditional fields of biochemistry, cell biology, and molecular biology. As the former fields mature, however, this phenomenon may not continue. As more tenure-track faculty positions are filled and these scientists obtain funding, the number of graduate students and postdoctoral scientists in the field will increase significantly, thereby increasing the competition for future positions. An increase in the size of the field could also make it more difficult for junior scientists to establish a reputation based on work performed within a project rather than on the number of publications with primary authorship. It is just that sort of reputation for personal scientific achievement that has always been critical for scientists in such fields as high-energy physics, in which publications include many authors listed in alphabetical order, but the field is small enough for the main players to recognize the relative contributions of the various participants. Even in that field, however, postdoctoral fellows and junior scientists have struggled to establish careers in their discipline, dealing with many of the same issues described here for life scientists (Glanz, 1998; American Institute of Physics, 1992).

SUMMARY

Little effort has been devoted to studying the impact of large-scale research on the career paths of life scientists. Without such an analysis, it is difficult to determine whether changes are needed. This lack of assessment is due in large part to a dearth of outcome data for trainees in biomedical science. NIH could fill this gap by expanding its capacity to track the career trajectories of trainees supported by any type of NIH funds and to assess their training environment.

Despite the paucity of such information, a number of potential obstacles in the career paths of scientists associated with large-scale research can be postulated now by examining trends in the field as a whole. Life scientists, both M.D.s and Ph.D.s, are struggling to establish traditional academic tenure-track careers in biomedical research, albeit for different reasons. Although a variety of other career options, including jobs in industry, are available to scientists, academic training programs generally are not geared toward those career paths, and students may find it difficult to obtain the information and mentoring needed to move in those directions. There are also a growing number of non-tenure-track positions in academia, but the traditional academic culture often does not provide the same degree of respect or compensation to scientists in these positions. In the case of M.D. scientists, the increasing demands of clinical practice and the burden of indebtedness from medical training are pushing would-be researchers into other career paths.

If large-scale projects are deemed worthy of substantial sums of federal support, they also clearly warrant the highest-caliber scientists and staff to perform and oversee the work. But if qualified scientists are expected to participate in such undertakings, they must have sufficient incentives to take on the risks and responsibilities involved. Trainees need adequate breadth of training and ample opportunity to establish a reputation for scientific achievement. Scientists in more senior positions need adequate remuneration, respect, and recognition for their work, whether it is independent or collaborative in nature. M.D.s need protected time to establish a successful career in research. Universities and NIH need work together to address these issues if large-scale projects are to be considered a valued component of the federal research portfolio.

One way to protect trainees from getting lost in the shuffle of a large-scale project is through funding-agency policies that regulate the staffing of the projects they support. For example, NIH could require principal investigators to describe the training value of project proposals that include trainee stipends in the budget. Indeed, NIH has already used this approach. The National Institute of General Medical Sciences (NIGMS) Protein Structure Initiative, which involves extensive data collection with limited hypothesis-driven research, strongly discourages the use of graduate students and postdoctoral scientists by requiring applicants to justify requests for their involvement and salary support. Instead, applicants are expected to include salary support for project managers and technicians.

NIH and universities could also do more to provide incentives for scientists who choose to work on large-scale collaborative projects. For example, NIH could be more flexible with regard to providing competitive salaries for scientific managers of large-scale projects. NIH could also develop more-detailed policies regarding publication and authorship for large-scale projects undertaken with its support. Universities could revise their policies on tenure and promotion to recognize the value of contributions made to collaborative projects. To accomplish this, academia may need to define new faculty and staff categories that better reflect the diversity in the types of research now being undertaken, along with appropriate criteria for performance evaluation and promotion. Universities could also expand their training programs to include such topics as management training for students and postdoctoral scientists who plan to work on large-scale projects. Given the changing nature of biomedical science, collaborative endeavors are likely to become more commonplace. Thus, it would be very beneficial to the field to nurture young scientists who wish to take these positions and learn the necessary skills to manage such projects.

7

Intellectual Property and Access to Research Tools and Data

S cientific research often leads to the generation of intellectual property—a term used to refer to a wide range of rights associated with inventions, discoveries, writings, product designs, and other creative works (Eisenberg, 1997). In recent years, the assignment and use of intellectual property rights have become more common in biomedical research, in some cases generating considerable controversy in the process. Patents in particular have been a recurrent cause for debate because of their potential effects on the dissemination and use of new knowledge, and thus on the progress of science. This issue may be especially salient for large-scale, collaborative projects that generate research tools[1] and products that may be useful to a large number of scientists in the field. Intellectual property issues may also be especially contentious for large-scale projects because providing a few scientists or institutions with very large amounts of money to conduct a large-scale project and then also rewarding them with many revenue-generating patents on the products of the research could be viewed as unfair.

The patent system is intended to promote innovation by rewarding inventors with the right to exclude others from using the invention in ex-

---

[1] The term "research tool" is defined as any discovery or invention that can facilitate or be used in subsequent research, including such things as reagents, devices, and databases. However, this term is not found in patent law, and no legal consequences arise from designating a particular discovery as a research tool.

change for an "enabling disclosure"[2] of the invention. (For definitions of terms associated with intellectual property, see Box 7-1). For the system to be successful, patents must restrict rights to products that are valuable and unlikely to be obtained by other means. This can be accomplished through the imposition of threshold requirements, such as novelty and utility.

Patents are generally thought to promote technological progress in two ways: by providing an economic incentive to devise new inventions and develop them into commercial products, and by promoting disclosure of new inventions to the public (Eisenberg, 1997). In the absence of patents, competitive forces encourage inventors to protect their ideas by keeping their inventions secret. Such an environment can lead to duplication of effort and reinvention because scientists are not aware of the advances of competitors. In contrast, if patent protection is available, scientists may learn more easily of advances in the field, allowing them to focus their energies on developing a subsequent invention (Thorner, 1997). However, scientists may have incentives for both withholding and disclosing research results (see Box 7-2), and disclosure need not necessarily take the form of a patent. The traditional method of scientific disclosure in the academic world has been simply through publication in peer-reviewed journals, rather than through patents.

Numerous developments over the last two decades—including increased commercial interest in the field and changes in federal policy to encourage patenting the results of government-sponsored research—have contributed to the increasing significance of intellectual property in biomedical research (National Research Council, 1997). In 1980, in an effort to promote commercial development of new technologies initiated by small businesses and nonprofit organizations, Congress passed legislation that uniformly[3] encouraged patenting of discoveries arising from federally supported research and promoted their commercial utilization (see Box 7-3). Although the Bayh-Dole Act targeted primarily small businesses rather than universities, the number of university-based patents has since increased greatly. The largest portion of the increase in university patenting has been in the biomedical sciences (National Research Council, 1997).

---

[2] Until 1999, when Congress amended the Patent Law, U.S. patent applications were not published. Disclosure, through publication of the patent, occurred only after the patent had been granted. In 1999, Congress passed an amendment to the U.S. Patent Law requiring the publication of most patent applications 18 months after filing, similar to the long-standing requirement abroad.

[3] Previously, universities could use Institutional Patent Agreements to take title of intellectual property generated with federal funding. However, agreements had to be negotiated on a case-by-case basis, and they varied across federal agencies. The new legislation established a uniform policy across federal agencies.

BOX 7-1   Terms Associated with Intellectual Property

Patents: The intent of the patent system is to promote innovation by rewarding inventors with a limited exclusivity on their discoveries in exchange for an "enabling disclosure" of the invention. A patent gives its owner the right to exclude all others from making, using, selling, or offering to sell the invention. The U.S. Patent Act authorizes patent protection for "any new and useful process, machine, manufacture, or composition of matter, or any new and useful improvement thereof," provided that the invention is new, useful, and nonobvious in light of the "prior art" (previous knowledge in the field as reflected primarily in publications and other patents).

Research exemption: Researchers are allowed an experimental-use exemption from licensing of patented inventions. A growing number of patents are issued on basic technology, especially in the field of biotechnology, where most of the value lies in the research potential to lead to subsequent innovations. Most European countries and Japan have included the principle of research exemption in their patent statues, but the U.S. Patent Act has not.

Exclusive versus nonexclusive licenses: A patent license is a contract between the owner of a patent and an independent party that wishes to make, use, or sell the invention claimed in the patent. Such a contract is essentially a promise by the patent owner that the owner will not sue the licensee for patent infringement, given compliance with the terms of the contract. A patented invention may be licensed exclusively to a single company, or nonexclusively to as many licensees as are interested and willing to negotiate terms.

Reach-through licensing: Patent holders reserve rights to future discoveries facilitated by use of their inventions. This is a commonly expressed concern regarding licensing strategies for research tools.

Patent pool: The term denotes the aggregation of intellectual property rights that are the subject of cross-licensing. It is an agreement between two or more patent holders to license their patents to each other or to third parties. A patent pool allows interested parties to gather all the tools needed to practice a certain technology in one place ("one-stop shopping") rather than obtaining licenses from each patent owner individually.

SOURCES: U.S. Patent Act, 35 U. S. § Code 101-103, 112; Clark et al. (2000); Ducor (1997).

Prior to 1980, the federal government sponsored primarily basic or "upstream" research, and broad, unpatented dissemination of results in the public domain was the norm for universities (Heller and Eisenberg, 1998). Fewer than 250 U.S. patents were issued to universities each year.[4] As a result, patents belonged almost exclusively to industry, where scientists

---

[4] See <http://www.autm.net/index_ie.html>.

BOX 7-2   Incentives for Disclosing and Withholding the Results of Scientific Research

Reasons for disclosing research results

- To obtain scientific recognition and credibility
- To facilitate widespread dissemination and use
- To defeat potential patent claims by others

Reasons for withholding research results

- To retain exclusive access for customers
- To avoid disclosure to rivals
- To preserve future patent rights

SOURCE: Eisenberg (2000).

---

and engineers were doing product-oriented "applied" research. Most patented innovations were incorporated into finished or near-market products and processes, because only then were they considered to be worth the costs associated with obtaining and protecting a patent. The new legislation, combined with the advent of biotechnology, has been a factor in changing this scenario and has contributed to a blurring of traditional distinctions between basic and applied research. Nonprofit institutions are now much more likely to patent their discoveries. In recent years, U.S, patents being issued to universities have exceeded 3,000 per year, with more than 3,700[5] issued to Universities in the year 2000 (Pressman, 2002). Nonprofit institutions now often pursue avenues of research that are similar to those in private industry, and research collaborations between industry and academic institutions are now widespread as well. Furthermore, many biotechnology companies have their origins in university-based research (Ducor, 1997). In fact, commercial biotechnology firms have attempted to fill a niche in research and development somewhere between the traditional basic science of academic laboratories and the targeted product development of pharmaceutical firms (Heller and Eisenberg, 1998).

The privatization of upstream biomedical research has led to intellectual property claims on research results that, in an earlier era, would have been made freely available in the public domain (Heller and Eisenberg, 1998). Indeed, many biotechnology patents are considered research tools rather than traditional end products, since they are useful primarily for

---

[5] This total, representing 2.4 percent of all utility patents issued in the year 2000, is the aggregate figure for 190 institutions.

BOX 7-3   Federal Technology Law

In 1980, Congress passed the Bayh-Dole Act* and the Stevenson-Wydler Technology Innovation Act.** Together, these acts allowed government contractors, small businesses, and nonprofit organizations to retain certain patent rights in government-sponsored research and permitted the funded entity to transfer the technology to third parties.

The stated intent of Bayh-Dole is to promote the commercialization and public availability of inventions made in the United States. The act permits recipients of federal grants and contracts to elect title to patentable "subject inventions" developed with the use of federal funds. If recipients elect title, the act requires them to file patent applications, seek commercialization opportunities, and report back to the funding agency on efforts to obtain utilization of their inventions. Bayh-Dole effectively shifted federal policy from a position of putting the results of government-sponsored research directly into the public domain for use by all to a pro-patent position that stressed the need for intellectual property rights as an incentive for industry to undertake the costly investment necessary to bring new products to market. This policy shift was based on a belief that private entities, given the incentives of the patent system, would do a better job of commercializing inventions than could be done by federal agencies. The act for the first time established a largely uniform government-wide policy on the treatment of inventions developed during federally supported research and development (R&D).

Stevenson-Wydler is the basic federal technology law. A principal policy established by the act is that agencies should ensure the full use of the results of the nation's federal investment in R&D. Another is that the law requires federal laboratories to take an active role in the transfer of federally owned or originated technology to both state and local governments and the private sector. Stevenson-Wydler requires agencies to establish offices of research and technology applications at their federal laboratories, and to devote a percentage of their R&D budgets to technology transfer.

---

*Pub. Law No. 96-517, 6(a), 94 Stat. 3015, 3019-27 (1980).
**Pub. Law No. 96-480, 94 Stat. 2311 (1980).
SOURCE: Adapted from National Research Council (1997).

---

further scientific research. Most large-scale research projects, as defined in this report, also produce research tools. The term "research tool" is not found in patent law, and no legal consequences arise from designating a particular discovery as a research tool; nonetheless, some patents that fall into this category have been the most contentious with regard to their impact on the progress of science. But the key question relates to access to the research tools, rather than to whether the tools should be patented or not. There are many different ways to transfer patented technologies to other institutions, and the methods chosen can have a significant impact on the availability of research tools. A research project may require access to many research tools, and the costs and administrative burden can mount quickly if it is necessary for researchers to negotiate separate licenses for each of these tools.

NONEXCLUSIVE AND EXCLUSIVE LICENSING

There has been considerable debate over the strategies used by NIH and universities to disseminate patented technologies developed with federal funds. Ultimately, the value of a research tool is likely to be greatest when it is widely available to all researchers who can use it, but there is no universal agreement as to how broad dissemination is best achieved. Once a research tool has been patented, there is a wide spectrum of options for exercising the intellectual property rights associated with that patent. At one extreme is no protection of the patent, in which no effort is made to prevent infringement. In essence, such a strategy makes the discovery freely available to anyone, but precludes others from restricting access through a patent of their own. More commonly, patented research tools are licensed to another party for use in research or product development, or for purposes of sublicensing to others. A license may be exclusive with a single company or nonexclusive, in which case anyone willing to negotiate a contract may have access to the technology (see Box 7-1). At many major universities, it is now common for industry-sponsored research agreements to stipulate that while ownership of any resulting patents will be retained by the university, the sponsoring company will have a first option to an exclusive license. And with the increase in university-industry partnerships, this approach applies to more research than in the past years (Ducor, 1997). Although the Bayh-Dole Act does not specify a preference for either exclusive or nonexclusive licenses, it does mandate a preference for licensing to small firms. But because small companies, especially start-up businesses, may depend on exclusive rights to establish a competitive advantage and ensure access to high-risk capital, the law may indirectly encourage universities to grant exclusive licenses (Henry et al., 2002). However, many scholars have suggested that nonexclusive licenses are more effective in ensuring the development and broad use of new discoveries.

Examples exist to support both sides of the debate. The Cohen-Boyer patent on basic recombinant DNA technology is an early example of a nonexclusive licensing policy that led to modest pricing and wide distribution of the technology. The decision to negotiate a nonexclusive license was critical to the industry, as this technology has contributed enormously to subsequent development of commercial biotechnology (National Research Council, 1997; U.S. Patent and Trademark Office, 2000). On the other hand, the technology for DNA sequencing instruments developed and patented at Caltech was licensed exclusively to Applied Biosystems

Incorporated (ABI) at the company's insistence. The technology has since been broadly disseminated and is widely available to researchers, usually through core facilities at universities. ABI is currently the leader in the world market for DNA sequencers, but other companies still have important market shares (National Research Council, 1997).

One case in which an exclusive license has been widely criticized for restricting the use of a common research tool is that of the patented "oncomouse" (National Research Council, 1994b; Institute of Medicine, 1996; Marshall, 2002a). In the 1980s, Philip Leder and his colleagues at Harvard developed a transgenic mouse that overexpressed the oncogene c-myc and was thus prone to developing cancer. Harvard has been granted three related patents on this oncomouse, and all three have been licensed exclusively to DuPont. The first patent, granted in 1988, claims rights to all transgenic animals predisposed to cancer. Thus, any scientist studying a transgenic animal that is prone to cancer must obtain a license from DuPont for permission to use it, regardless of who created the particular transgenic mouse line or what cancer-related gene was altered in its germline.

In 2000, NIH brokered an agreement with DuPont in which the company agreed to provide a "free research license" to any NIH scientist or NIH grantee doing noncommercial studies with an oncomouse. However, scientists and their institutions must agree to the terms of the contract, which stipulate reach-through license agreements on the resultant downstream research (see the next section of this chapter). Anyone who wants to use an oncomouse in drug screening must obtain a commercial license and pay a considerable fee.

Some academic institutions have refused to sign a contract with DuPont, and many have suggested that the broad claims of the patent would not survive a court challenge; however, universities are reluctant to pursue costly litigation (Marshall, 2002a). The patents have already withstood legal challenges in Europe and Japan, but the Canadian Supreme Court recently ruled that the oncomouse is unpatentable in Canada.

Restricting the use of transgenic mice could greatly impede cancer research because such mice serve as basic research tools and models for human cancer and can also be used to screen for or test new therapeutics. Thus, DuPont's aggressive enforcement of the oncomouse patents could be an obstacle to achieving the goals of NCI's Mouse Models of Human Cancer Consortium (described in Chapter 3).

A recent survey of U.S. institutions holding gene sequence patents showed that companies and nonprofit organizations tend to favor different strategies for licensing their discoveries (Henry et al., 2002), perhaps reflecting different goals or stages of product development. For example, companies may have more end-stage products for which a nonexclusive license would generate the most revenue, while nonprofits may have more upstream products. Whatever the reason, private firms reported that an average of 27 percent of all licenses granted were exclusive, while nonprofits reported an average of 68 percent. An earlier survey of academic technology transfer executives showed that about 50 percent of licenses granted by universities were exclusive; in contrast only 22 percent of licenses granted by the NIH in 2001 were exclusive (Pressman, 2002).

NIH appears to favor the nonexclusive approach to licensing, given the set of rules it adopted in 1999 with the intent of promoting greater sharing of tools and new materials. The guidelines[6] for sharing research tools encompasses four principles:

- Scientists who receive federal funds must avoid agreements that stifle academic communications.
- Scientists should not seek or agree to exclusive licenses on research tools (defined as inventions whose "primary usefulness" is "discovery" and not a product to be approved by the Food and Drug Administration [FDA]).
- Academic scientists should "minimize administrative impediments" on exchanges of materials by refusing "unacceptable conditions" (such as reach-through provisions).
- Academic institutions should be as flexible in dealing with others (including companies) as they would have others be with them.

Perhaps not surprisingly, some smaller biotechnology companies, whose survival may depend on selling such research tools, are not enthusiastic about these guidelines (Marshall, 1999).

REACH-THROUGH LICENSE AGREEMENTS

One difficulty in licensing research tools is that the value of the license is impossible to determine in advance, so it can be difficult to define mutually agreeable license terms. One of the most contentious issues regarding the licensing of patented research tools is the "reach-through" clause. Reach-through license agreements (RTLAs) give the owner of a patented invention used in upstream stages of research rights in subsequent downstream discoveries. Such rights may take the form of a royalty on sales that result from use of the upstream research tool, an exclusive or nonexclusive license on future discoveries, or an option to acquire such a license. In principle, such agreements could offer advantages to both patent holders and the scientists who use the patented tools in their re-

---

[6] Guidelines available at <http://ott.od.nih.gov/NewPages/RTguide_final.html>.

search because they impose an obligation to share profits of successful research without adding to the costs of unsuccessful research. For example, RTLAs could allow scientists with limited funds to use tools and defer payment until the research yielded valuable results. Patent holders may also prefer a chance at larger payoffs from sales of downstream products, rather than certain but smaller up-front fees. In practice, however, companies fear that RTLAs may lead to stacked, overlapping, and inconsistent claims on potential downstream products. From their perspective, each RTLA royalty obligation becomes a prospective tax on sales of a new product, and the more research tools are used in developing a product, the higher the tax burden will be (Heller and Eisenberg, 1998; Eisenberg, 1997). RTLAs can also create challenges for universities, as scientists may find it more difficult to obtain research funding for projects in which they are entailed.

RESEARCH EXEMPTIONS

One potential way to prevent technology licenses from impeding the progress of scientific research is an experimental-use license exemption, or research exemption, for patented research tools. In principle, such an exemption allows scientists to use research tools without obtaining a license if the research is purely experimental and is not aimed at developing a patentable or marketable product. The goal of this exemption is to facilitate widespread use in subsequent research while preserving the financial interests of the patent holder. Most European countries and Japan have included the principle of research exemption in their patent statutes, but the U.S. Patent Act has not.[7] U.S. courts have recognized a research exemption in theory, but most court cases have arisen in instances in which the commercial stakes are high, and the exemption is unlikely to be sustained (Eisenberg, 1997). Unfortunately, it is difficult to define experimental use in such a way as to maintain the commercial value of research tools for the patent holder. According to Eisenberg (1997: 13):

> The problem is that researchers are ordinary consumers of patented research tools, and that if these consumers were exempt from infringement liability, patent holders would have nowhere else to turn to collect

---

[7] Congress has enacted laws for two specific research use exceptions. The first permits basic research on an invention during the life of a patent if the research is to develop and submit information to FDA (the Drug Price Competition and Patent Term Restoration Act, 35 U.S.C., Section 271[e]). The second permits the use and reproduction of a protected plant variety for plan breeding or other bona fide research (Plant Variety Protection Act, 7 U.S.C. 2321 et seq., Section 2544).

patent royalties. Another way of looking at the problem is that one firm's research tool may be another firm's end product. This is particularly likely in contemporary molecular biology, in which research is big business and there is money to be made by developing and marketing research tools for use by other firms. An excessively broad research exemption could eliminate incentives for private firms to develop and disseminate new research tools, which could on balance do more harm than good to the research enterprise.

Furthermore, some industry executives have noted that although industry previously often gave university research a de facto research exemption, they are now often more reluctant to do so because in many cases, university researchers are seen as competing directly with their own research.[8] As a result, companies may feel burdened by the requirement to license the results of university research that have been patented (but formerly would have been freely available) when the universities continue to expect an exemption for use of the companies' patented research tools.

A recent court ruling[9] may also make it more difficult for universities to a claim research exemption if they are sued for patent infringement. In ordering a district court to reevaluate its decision in an infringement case brought against Duke University, a U.S. Court of Appeals for the Federal Circuit found that the district court had applied an overly broad concept of the very narrow and strictly limited experimental-use defense (Ergenzinger and Spruill, 2003). In ruling against Duke, the appeals court stated that even if a university is pursuing research "with no commercial application whatsoever," the institution should not presume that its actions automatically qualify as an exception to infringement.

Duke had argued that its use of patented laboratory equipment did not constitute infringement because the equipment was used under the authority of a government research grant and was covered by an exception for experimental uses. However, the scientist claiming infringement offered the counter argument that Duke is in the business of obtaining grants and developing possible commercial applications for the fruits of its academic research, and therefore the research exemption should not apply.

Previous court rulings have established that the experimental-use exception can be claimed only for actions performed for amusement, to satisfy idle curiosity, or for strictly philosophical inquiry. The defense

---

[8] Personal communication with Richard Nelson, School of International and Public Affairs, Columbia University.

[9] *Madey v. Duke University*, USCAFC, 01-1567. Decided October 3, 2002.

does not apply when the use is undertaken "in the guise of scientific inquiry" or in furtherance of a party's legitimate business. The new appellate ruling states that in the case of a major research university such as Duke, such business includes research that educates students and faculty members, attracts additional grants, and helps "increase the status of the institution and lure lucrative research grants, students, and faculty." Several major research universities are now petitioning the Supreme Court to review the decision because they believe it will hinder research by forcing scientists to obtain permission before using patented technologies (Malakoff, 2003).

PATENT POOLS

Perhaps a more viable approach to reducing potential licensing obstacles associated with research tools is to establish patent pools. Over the last 150 years, patent pools have played an important role in shaping other fields, such as the automobile, aircraft, and telecommunications industries. These patent pools have emerged, sometimes with the help of government, when licenses under multiple patent rights have been necessary to develop important new products (Heller and Eisenberg, 1998; U.S. Patent and Trademark Office, 2000). A patent pool is an agreement between two or more patent holders to license their patents to each other or to third parties. In theory, this type of arrangement can simplify research and reduce transaction costs by allowing interested parties to gather all the tools needed to practice with a certain technology in one place ("one-stop shopping") rather than obtaining licenses from each patent owner individually (see Box 7-4). Patent pools can also facilitate information exchange and the distribution of risks associated with research and development. But patent pools can also potentially have detrimental effects (see Box 7-4). For example, a patent pool could theoretically shield invalid patents, eliminate competition, and inflate prices.

Patent pools can also conflict with antitrust laws that were designed to prevent the creation of monopolies and restraints on interstate commerce (U.S. Patent and Trademark Office, 2000). As a result, the Department of Justice evaluated all patent pools prior to the 1960s and created a list of patent licensing practices that were per se antitrust violations. More recently, the Department of Justice and the Federal Trade Commission (FTC) have recognized that patent pools can have significant procompetitive effects and may also improve a business' ability to survive in a time of rapid technological innovation in a global economy. In 1995, the Department of Justice and the FTC issued Antitrust Guidelines for the Licensing of Intellectual Property and set forth enforcement policies (see Box 7-5). These guidelines can be summarized in two broad questions:

BOX 7-4   Potential Benefits and Risks of Patent Pooling

Potential Benefits

- Elimination of problems caused by "blocking" patents or "stacking" licenses
- Significant reduction of licensing transaction costs and litigation
- Distribution of risks associated with research and development
- Institutionalized exchange of technical information not covered by patents (reduction in trade secrets)

Potential Risks

- Inflation of the costs of competitively priced goods
- Shielding of invalid patents
- Elimination of competition by encouraging collusion and price fixing

---

SOURCE: Clark et al. (2000).

- Is the proposed licensing program likely to integrate complementary patent rights?
- If so, are the resulting competitive benefits likely to outweigh the competitive harm posed by other aspects of the program?

The recent formation of patent pools in a number of fields suggests that the social and economic benefits of these arrangements can outweigh their costs (U.S. Patent and Trademark Office, 2000). Patent pools could offer similar potential benefits to the field of biotechnology, serving the interests of both the public and private industry by eliminating patent stacks and licensing bottlenecks. In the case of biomedical research, however, the obstacles to establishing patent pools may be greater than in other fields. Because patents are often particularly important to the pharmaceutical and biotechnology industries, firms may be less willing to participate in patent pools that undermine the gains of exclusivity (Levin et al., 1987). For example, it can be more difficult to "invent around" gene or protein patents than the device or process patents that are more common in other industries. Conflicting agendas of the various patent holders and their tendency to overvalue their contribution to the pool can also make it difficult to reach mutually satisfactory agreements or to develop standard license terms. Patents on research tools are likely to include a diverse set of techniques, reagents, sequences, and instruments, making it difficult to compare the value of the various patents in a potential pool. This heterogeneity is complicated by the fact that licensing agreements are likely to be negotiated early in the course of research and develop-

BOX 7-5   Patent Pool Guidelines in the Antitrust Guidelines for
the Licensing of Intellectual Property (issued by the Federal
Trade Commission and the U.S. Department of Justice in 1995)

Intellectual property pooling is procompetitive when it:

- Integrates complementary technologies.
- Reduces transaction costs.
- Clears blocking positions.
- Avoids costly infringement litigation.
- Promotes the dissemination of technology.

Excluding firms from an intellectual property pool may be anticompetitive if:

- The excluded firms cannot compete effectively in the relevant market for the good incorporating the licensed technologies.
- The pool participants collectively possess market power in the relevant market.
- The limitations on participation are not reasonably related to the efficient development and exploitation of the pooled technologies.

Patents pools must meet the following criteria for approval:

- The patents in the pool must be valid and not expired.
- There must be no aggregation of competitive technologies and setting a single price for them.
- An independent expert should be used to determine whether a patent is essential to complement technologies in the pool.
- The pool agreement must not disadvantage competitors in downstream product markets.
- The pool participants must not collude on prices outside the scope of the pool, e.g., on downstream products.

SOURCE: Clark et al. (2000); U.S. Department of Justice and Federal Trade Commission (1995) (see <http://www.usdoj.gov/atr/public/guidelines/ipguide.htm>).

ment, when the outcome is uncertain and the value of downstream products is unknown (Heller and Eisenberg, 1998).

UNIVERSITY POLICIES AND TECHNOLOGY TRANSFER OFFICES

Regardless of what approach is taken to licensing patented innovations, perhaps one of the key issues in fostering the development of technologies developed at universities with federal funding lies in the policies and strategies used by universities to disseminate their innovations and to capitalize on their patented intellectual property. A major intent of the laws that encourage universities to patent the results of federally funded research is to facilitate technology transfer for further research and development. But patents also provide universities with opportunities for new revenue sources with none of the restrictions that may be associated with traditional funding sources. Optimizing technology transfer to promote the commercialization of discoveries and maximizing licensing revenues may entail different strategies; thus the policies of universities regarding intellectual property rights should be considered carefully, within the context of their academic values and mission to advance knowledge.

Since 1980, NIH and many universities have created technology transfer offices to patent and license their discoveries for further development. Protection of intellectual property rights has helped researchers and institutions generate research funding and has also helped new biotechnology firms raise investment capital and pursue product development (National Research Council, 1997). A recent survey conducted by the Association of University Technology Managers (AUTM) found that the adjusted gross income received by universities from licenses and options was $1.26 billion in 2000. The survey also found that at least 454 new companies were created and 347 products were made commercially available that year based on academic discoveries (Pressman, 2002). However, these numbers must be placed in proper perspective. Despite the perception of many that the role of technology transfer offices is to generate revenue for research, university-based technology is generally not very lucrative, except for a few of the most prominent research institutions. Data from the AUTM survey consistently document that gross revenues generated from a university's patent licensing activity average approximately 4 percent of the research dollars spent by that institution (net revenues are even less after the administrative and legal costs of the technology transfer activity have been paid). Furthermore, few campuses benefit from patents for "blockbuster" products. Of the reported 20,968 active licenses in fiscal year 2000, only 125 (0.6 percent) generated more than $1,000,000 in royalty income (Pressman, 2002).[10]

Thus, it may be beneficial to the public for universities to consider a variety of patenting and licensing alternatives that may yield lower revenues but ensure wider public use. For example, for a given patent, an exclusive license might generate the most revenue or might be the fastest way to generate income, but such a license might not necessarily be the best strategy for fostering the most downstream research activity. In some instances, the objectives of the Bayh-Dole Act might also be achieved by making patented university research results available to all who want to use them at a very low transaction cost.

---

[10] By comparison, revenues of $100,000/year are roughly equivalent to increasing a university's endowment by $3 million, assuming a 3 percent rate of interest.

Further research is needed to determine whether the frequent inclination of universities to license out their patented inventions exclusively is warranted by the need to stimulate investment in downstream product development or whether exclusive licensing has simply become a default method for transferring technology to industry (Henry et al., 2002). If the latter is true, NIH could facilitate access to research results on a case-by-case basis by specifying broad licensing expectations whenever feasible in issuing program announcement (PAs) or requests for applications (RFAs) for new initiatives.

EXAMPLES OF INTELLECTUAL PROPERTY AND DATA SHARING ISSUES ASSOCIATED WITH LARGE-SCALE PROJECTS

Genomics and DNA Patents

Debates regarding patents on DNA sequences and access to sequence data have been frequent and often quite contentious in recent years. Although raw DNA sequences are viewed as "products of nature" and are therefore not patentable, purified and isolated DNA sequences are now routinely patented. Such DNA sequences are considered large chemical compounds that may be patented as "compositions of matter" under the same principles previously applied to smaller molecules.

The number of DNA-based patents issued per year increased exponentially between 1980 and 1998. In 1999 the number leveled off, and in 2000 the number began to decrease for the first time (see Figure 7-1). During the brief history of genomics research, the public and private strategies for publication and patenting of DNA sequences have varied and often overlapped, at times favoring patent applications, with or without pursuing patent protection, and at times using rapid publication to disclose findings (Eisenberg, 2000; see Box 7-6). Indeed, although about half the patents are held by for-profit companies, the U.S. Government holds more patents on DNA sequences than any single private firm or institution (see Figures 7-2 and 7-3). From an international perspective, the vast majority of DNA-based patents are assigned to owners based in the United States (see Figure 7-4). Between 1980 and 1993, 80 percent of DNA patents were based in this country. The next-largest holder of patents was Japan, with 7 percent of the total. All other countries held less than 3 percent.

The most significant obstacles to obtaining patent protection for DNA sequences have been the utility requirement, which limits protection to inventions that have a demonstrated practical use, and the disclosure requirements, which limit the scope of allowable claims (Eisenberg, 1997). In fact, these issues have been at the heart of the debate surrounding

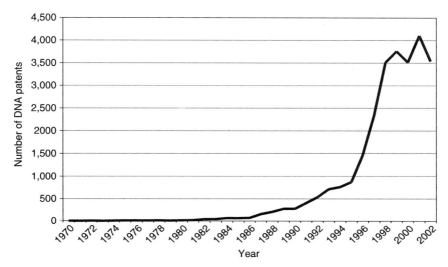

FIGURE 7-1   DNA-based U.S. patents, 1970–2002.
SOURCE: LeRoy Walters (<http://www.stanford.edu/class/siw198q/websites/genomics>) and DNA Patent Database (<www.genomic.org>).

patent applications for gene fragments known as expressed sequence tags (ESTs) (see Chapter 3), which are often accompanied by few data regarding the biological function of the sequence beyond what can be hypothesized from comparisons with similar sequences with known function. This situation led the U.S. Patent and Trademark Office to adjust its utility standards in 2000, essentially making the requirements for DNA sequences more stringent (Kyd, 2000).

Even in the case of full-length genes, however, patents can generate controversy. Most often, discovery of a disease-associated gene first leads to the development of a diagnostic test. If patent holders choose to enforce their patent rights aggressively, they can preclude scientists and physicians from testing patients in their own laboratories, which leads to increased costs. Such was the case for the breast cancer-related genes BRCA1 and BRCA2. In other instances, such as Canavan's[11] disease, the tests could be performed locally but only after paying a royalty for each test that was performed, again leading to higher costs. In the latter example, the issue was especially contentious because patient advocacy groups had been very involved in collecting patient DNA samples that were used to identify the gene. They then found that access to the resultant diagnos-

---

[11] Canavan's disease is a progressive, degenerative disorder of the central nervous system. It develops in infancy, usually between the ages of 3 and 9 months. Death usually occurs within 18 months after onset of symptoms.

BOX 7-6 Examples of Intellectual Property Strategies for Large-Scale Projects

The SNP Consortium: The overall objective is (1) to maximize the number of single nucleotide polymorphisms (SNPs) that enter the public domain at the earliest possible date, and (2) to be free of third-party encumbrances such that the map can be used by all without financial or other intellectual property obligations. To meet objective (2), the SNP Consortium intends to withhold public release of identified SNPs until mapping has been achieved to prevent facilitating the patenting of the same SNPs by third parties. Mapped SNPs will be publicly released quarterly, approximately one quarter after they have been identified. The intellectual property plan is intended to maintain the priority dates of discovery of the unmapped SNPs during the period between identification and release, for use as "prior art."

The National Human Genome Research Institute (NHGRI) policy on release of human genome sequence data: In NHGRI's opinion, the raw human genomic DNA sequence, in the absence of additional demonstrated biological information, lacks demonstrated specific utility and therefore is an inappropriate material for patent filing. NIH is concerned that patent application on large blocks of primary human genomic DNA sequence could have a chilling effect on the development of future inventions of useful products. NHGRI will monitor grantee activity in this area to determine whether attempts are being made to patent large blocks of primary human genomic DNA sequence.

The Bermuda Rules: An agreement entered into at the International Strategy Meeting on Human Genome Sequencing, held in Bermuda in 1996, states that "all human genomic sequence information, generated by centers funded for large-scale human sequencing, should be freely available and in the public domain in order to encourage research and development and to maximize its benefit to society." The Bermuda Rules have been criticized for promoting public disclosure of data that have not been checked for accuracy.

SOURCE: Adapted from Eisenberg (2000).

---

tic test was hindered by the licensing policy of Miami Children's Hospital, the gene patent holder (Marshall, 2000). As a result of such cases, legislation has been proposed that would exempt researchers and clinicians who use genetic-based diagnostic tests from patent infringement—similar to legislation enacted in 1996 exempting doctors from suits for using patented medical or surgical procedures (Boahene, 2002). The Biotechnology Industry Organization opposes such legislation on the grounds that it would devastate the biotechnology industry and drive investors to other industries (Warner, 2002).

A related controversial issue regarding DNA patents hinges on the level of effort and inventiveness associated with such discoveries. The

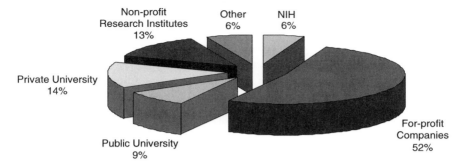

FIGURE 7-2   U.S. DNA-based patent assignees.
SOURCE: Stephen McCormack and Robert Cook-Deegan, (<http://www.stanford.edu/class/siw198q/websites/genomics/entry.htm>) and DNA Patent Database (<www.genomic.org>), August 1999.

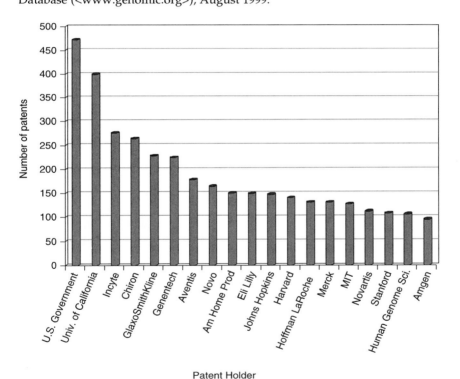

FIGURE 7-3   Number of patents in the DNA Patent Database assigned to various entities in academia, industry, and government, 1980–1999.
SOURCE: Robert Cook-Deegan (<http://www.stanford.edu/class/siw198q/websites/genomics/entry.htm>) and DNA Patent Database (<www.genomic.org>), December 1999.

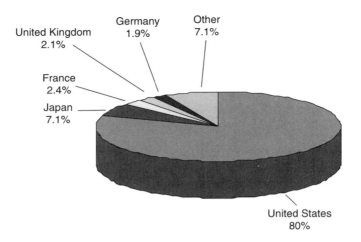

FIGURE 7-4   Ownership (assignee country) of 1028 DNA-based patents 1980–1993. SOURCE: Stephen McCormack and Robert Cook-Deegan (<http://www. stanford. edu/class/siw198q/websites/genomics/entry.htm>) and DNA Patent Database, (<www.genomic.org>), August 1999.

patentability of a novel DNA sequence depends on the absence of disclosure of structurally similar DNA molecules rather than on the level of inventive skill necessary to obtain the sequence. Research scientists may view this as incompatible with the traditional perceptions of scientific achievement. And by simply identifying a gene sequence, a patent holder can claim broad rights to future treatments that target the gene product. Indeed, if patent law systematically allocates stronger rights to those who identify novel DNA sequences while withholding effective patent protection from those who undertake the more difficult tasks of elucidating gene function and developing new therapies, it stands to reason that the latter two activities will be less lucrative than the business of identifying novel DNA sequences (Eisenberg, 1997). There is currently little hard evidence that this scenario is being played out, and in fact, firms that own the sequence patents will still undoubtedly be motivated to learn the functions of those genes. However, narrowing the scope of patents on biotechnology innovations that are still far removed from clinical application might stimulate a broader range of research activity by more institutions, and thus lead to better therapeutics in the long run. Many questions remain regarding the potential strength and value of patents that cover related subjects, such as proteins that are coded by patented DNA sequences, as is discussed further in the next section.

Protein Patents

Analysis of the human genome sequence has led to the conclusion that the genome may contain significantly fewer genes than the previous estimate of 100,000. Although current methods for identifying functional protein coding sequences may underestimate the actual number of genes, recent estimates suggest that there are fewer than 50,000 (Lander et al., 2001; Venter et al., 2001). Nonetheless, researchers speculate that there may be as many as 2 million different proteins, suggesting that many variant proteins can be produced from a single gene. The difference between the two numbers lies in alterations in DNA transcription and RNA splicing, as well as post-translational modifications of the protein products, all of which can have a profound influence on the function and activity of the resultant proteins. According to the U.S. Patent and Trademark Office, researchers can make separate patent claims on these variant proteins even if the parent gene is already patented, as long as the identified changes lead to new and unclaimed functions and uses. The result could potentially be a confusing landscape of competing gene and protein patent claims, perhaps setting the stage for legal battles for control over further research and development. This may be especially true if a protein variant shows a stronger correlation with disease than is the case for the earlier gene that was patented (Service, 2001b). To avoid the possibility of expensive litigation, companies may find themselves cross-licensing many related patented discoveries. On the other hand, some companies are hoping to develop ways of circumventing the claims of genomics companies that have patent rights for making proteins from patented gene sequences in bacteria. For example, GeneProt, a new proteomics firm, plans to synthesize proteins chemically (Service, 2001a).

Many companies appear to be banking on the patentability and profitability of identifying and characterizing unique protein variants. Dozens of new biotechnology firms have emerged in the past few years either to conduct large-scale searches for proteins (proteomics) or to sell research tools to those doing the searching. Most pharmaceutical companies have also launched their own proteomics efforts. All are now racing to find and patent as many proteins as possible. One of the leading companies intended to file 4,000 patents on proteins whose functions are known and linked to disease by the end of 2001. Investors also initially appeared to have confidence in the profitability of this approach. Proteomics companies attracted more than $530 million in venture capital funds in 2000 and 2001, and stock offerings have raised hundreds of millions more (Service, 2001c). More recently, however, investment in proteomics companies has declined because of predictions of lower profitability (Warner, 2002).

Because of all the competing efforts, many proteomics researchers are concerned that all the data will be locked up by various private companies. As a result, there is great interest in undertaking publicly funded proteomics projects whose results would be deposited and organized in a freely accessible database. In October 2001, scientific leaders in the field met with representatives of NIH and other government funding agencies, as well as proteomics companies, to discuss launching a coordinated initiative, perhaps modeled after the NIH-funded Alliance for Cell Signaling (see Chapter 3). The group recommended pilot projects in three areas—profiling protein expression in selected tissues, detailing proteins' functions, and creating new bioinformatics tools (Service, 2001c).

Databases

With the recent increase in large-scale biomedical research projects that generate immense datasets have come concerns about the organization and accessibility of databases. To optimize the progress of science, scientists may have to combine data from a variety of academic and commercial sources, but this data aggregation can present a serious obstacle for both technical and proprietary reasons. A lack of uniformity or standardization in quality control can be a serious impediment to combining data from different sources. Attempts to protect the intellectual property value of data add additional challenges. Over the past 5 years, both academic and commercial biologists have attempted to use "pass-through" rights that place restrictions on data even after they have been incorporated into other databases. This practice creates opportunities for gridlock. But biotechnology companies in particular worry about making a large financial commitment to a project if there is a risk that the underlying data could belong to someone else. U.S. companies have resorted to a sophisticated assortment of strategies to prevent copying, including contracts, download restrictions, and frequent updates. At the other end of the spectrum, the "open source code" model that was used to develop free computer software was discussed as an option for the public databases containing human genome sequences, although that strategy was ultimately rejected (Sulston and Ferry, 2002). In such a model, anyone could freely use the information in the database to conduct research, to develop products, or to redistribute the information in any form. However, anyone who did so would not be allowed to place new restrictions on further development or redistribution of the data.

Intellectual property law in the United States does not cover databases. Recently, however, the concept of database protection has been discussed frequently, in part as the result of a 1996 directive from the

European community to its members to create in Europe a new type of database that restricts use of the information. In fact, several unsuccessful attempts have been made to pass similar legislation in the United States since that directive was issued (Maurer et al., 2001). Although the European approach has been offered as a model to address the complex issues of database access and use, the legislation is actually unlikely to alter the strategies currently used to protect databases. In fact, critics have argued that the European Community directive has eroded the public domain, overprotected synthetic data of doubtful value (e.g., telephone numbers), and raised new barriers to data aggregation (Maurer et al., 2001). The threshold requirements of the directive have proven to be quite low, and most lawsuits have been brought by a small number of companies that create synthetic data, in essence making such data more valuable than genuine information.

A recent report of the National Research Council (1999) examines trends in access to scientific databases and makes recommendations for striking a balance between legitimate rights to protection and open access for the public good. A symposium hosted by the National Academies in 2002 further examined the potential negative effects of a diminishing public domain for scientific data, caused in part by pressures to commercialize and legislative efforts to protect intellectual property rights (Jenkins, 2002b).

Patient Confidentiality and Consent

Many of the theoretical large-scale projects described in chapter 2, as well as many of the ongoing projects described in chapter 3, entail the collection and analysis of human samples. As such, these endeavors require additional considerations with regard to data access and research on human subjects. There is an inherent tension in biomedical research between the need to protect the confidentiality of individuals and the need for access to information in order to make progress in understanding and treating disease. Because the data collected in large-scale projects are often placed in publicly accessible databases, considerations of privacy, confidentiality, and informed consent must be taken into account before, during, and after the study.

A common approach to obtaining informed consent for the use of human samples in specimen banks is to develop a very general consent form that will allow future, unspecified research to be conducted without the need to reacquire consent for every subsequent study. However, such an approach may come into question if a future project entails such objectives as genetic analysis with linkage to health information or the inclusion of data in public databases, or even if the samples are shared more widely within the scientific community than was originally anticipated. Because of the potential for a breach of privacy and subsequent discrimination or other repercussions, great care must be taken to protect the identity of sample donors. The NCI has developed guidelines for protecting the identities of tissue donors while still maintaining links to data on clinical information,[12] but researchers and their institution are responsible for protecting human subjects in studies carried out under their purview.

The tremendous concern about patient confidentiality in the United States is due in part to both hypothetical and actual lapses in the routine practice of medicine—for example, the management of the medical records in the ordinary setting of day-to-day hospital business, or the misuse of patient information by health care insurers. However, recent legislation aimed at redressing such lapses could also affect researchers' access to patient samples. Known as HIPAA, or the Health Insurance Portability and Accountability Act, the legislation contains rules that protect individually identifiable health information (Box 7-7). Because the enforcement of the rules will only begin in April of 2003, the impact of HIPAA on biomedical research is not yet known, but there is great concern within the biomedical scientific community.

EFFECTS OF INTELLECTUAL PROPERTY CLAIMS ON THE SHARING OF DATA AND RESEARCH TOOLS

Although concerns have been raised that intellectual property claims could inhibit access to data and research tools, little quantitative assessment has been undertaken to determine whether those concerns are valid. However, a survey of academic life scientists undertaken in 1997 found that 20 percent of respondents had delayed publication of their research results by more than 6 months at least once in the last 3 years to allow for patent application, to protect their scientific lead, to slow the dissemination of undesired results, to allow time to negotiate a patent, or to resolve disputes over the ownership of intellectual property (Blumenthal et al., 1997). Multivariate analysis indicated that participation in an academic-industry research relationship and engagement in the commercialization of university research were significantly associated with delays in publication. Notably, scientists who reported conducting research on goals similar to that of the Human Genome Project were also more likely to

---

[12] <http://www3.cancer.gov/confidentiality.html>.

BOX 7-7   Health Insurance Portability and Accountability Act (HIPAA)

The Health Insurance Portability and Accountability Act (HIPAA) of 1996 includes a clause known as the "Privacy Rule." The Privacy Rule is a federal regulation that governs the protection of individually identifiable health information. The Rule was enacted to increase the privacy protection of health information identifying individuals who are living or deceased, and to regulate known and unanticipated risks to privacy that may accompany the use and disclosure of personal health information. It is administered and enforced by the DHHS Office of Civil Rights (OCR). Those who must comply with the Privacy Rule must do so by April 14, 2003, except small health plans, which have an extra year to comply.

Research entities to which the Privacy Rule applies include health care clearinghouses, health plans, and health care providers that electronically transmit health information in connection with a transaction for which DHHS has adopted standards under HIPAA. The Rule may also affect researchers who obtain individually identifiable health information from covered entities through collaborative or contractual arrangements. Decisions about whether and how to implement the Privacy Rule reside with the researcher and his/her institution. The roles of several federal agencies regarding the Privacy Rule are described below:

- Office for Civil Rights (OCR): Oversight and civil enforcement responsibility for the Privacy Rule are under the auspices of OCR, DHHS.
- Department of Justice (DOJ): Enforcement of the criminal penalties for violations of the Privacy Rule is under the auspice of DOJ.
- National Institutes of Health (NIH): Development of educational materials for researchers, in collaboration with other DHHS research agencies, is the role of NIH. NIH is not involved in enforcing or monitoring compliance with the Privacy Rule.

SOURCE: NIH Guide: Impact of the HIPAA Privacy Rule on NIH processes involving the review, funding, and progress monitoring of grants, cooperative agreements and research contracts, February 5, 2003. See <http://grants1.nih.gov/grants/guide/notice-files/NOT-OD-03-025.html>.

---

deny requests for information, data, and materials than were other life scientists.

More recently, a survey focusing on geneticists[13] found that among those who had requested published data, materials, or techniques from another academician, 47 percent reported that at least one request was

---

[13]A stratified sample of 3,000 faculty members was selected. The sample included 219 grantees of the Human Genome Project and 1,547 faculty members in genetics or human genetics departments. The remainder of the sample (n = 1234) was randomly selected so that half came from nonclinical departments (n = 617) and half from clinical departments (n = 617).

denied[14] (Campbell et al., 2002). The requests most likely to be denied were for biomaterials such as mice or viruses (35 percent), followed by sequence data (28 percent), findings (25 percent), phenotypes (22 percent), and laboratory techniques (16 percent). Figure 7-5 shows the reasons given by geneticists for intentionally withholding from other scientists information, data, or materials concerning their own published research. A number of respondents reported that such withholding of data had adverse effects on their ability to reproduce the work of other investigators, on the timeliness of their own publications, and on their ability to pursue chosen research directions. These adverse effects on research progress at the individual and field levels were more likely to be reported by geneticists than by investigators who had experienced such withholding in other life science fields. Many geneticists indicated that the situation was having a negative impact on communication within their field, the education of young scientists, and the rate of scientific progress.

Even when data are placed into a publicly accessible database, conflicts over rights to and use of the data can arise (Marshall, 2002c; Roberts, 2002). For example, a group of collaborating scientists led by the Marine Biological Laboratory (MBL) in Woods Hole, Massachusetts, won a 5-year, $2.6 million award from NIH in 1997 to sequence the genome of a disease-causing protozoan. Because NIH required rapid availability of the data, raw sequence data were routinely posted on a public website. However, the group also posted guidelines that limited database users to reagent development or mutually agreed-upon projects. When two scientists published a paper that included analysis of data from a variety of public databases, including the MBL site, the MBL organizers protested and closed down the website. This is a relatively new issue associated with large-scale projects that generate databases for use by the scientific community. Traditionally, scientists are expected to share data and reagents following publication, but prior to publishing, scientists have had discretion in choosing what to share and with whom. However, NIH has required grantees to release data as soon as they are generated, often well before publication in peer-reviewed journals. This policy is designed to speed the pace of research and to allow the field as a whole to benefit from the large investment made to generate the data, but it clearly raises new questions regarding the data's use, analysis, and publication.

The advisory committee for the International Nucleotide Sequence Databases, which includes Genbank, recently endorsed a data sharing

---

[14]Respondents estimated that they had made an average of 8.8 requests for information, data, or materials regarding published research in the previous 3 years, with 10 percent of those requests being denied.

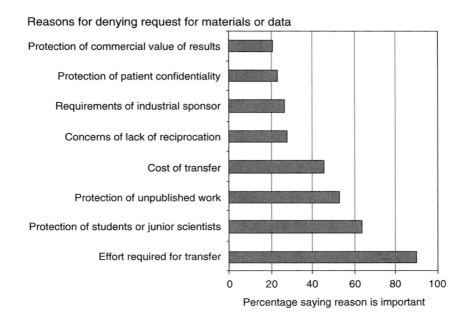

FIGURE 7-5   A survey of geneticists examined the reasons for which requests for data and materials were denied.
SOURCE: Campbell et al., 2002.

policy that specifically prohibits use or publication restrictions such as those described above, as well as licensing requirements (Brunak et al., 2002). A recent report of the National Research Council (2003) urges scientists, funding agencies, and publishers to adhere to a uniform policy for sharing data and reagents. Using the acronym UPSIDE (universal principle of sharing integral data expeditiously), the report reinforces an author's obligation to release data and materials quickly to allow others to verify or replicate published findings. New guidelines for sharing data are also being developed by NIH. For instance, the agency will expect investigators to include information in their research applications about how they plan to share the resultant data or why they are unable to do so (Spieler, 2002). But it is not clear how adherence to the guidelines will be monitored and enforced, or whether they will lead to real changes in behavior within the scientific community. In principle, NIH has numerous legal authorities available to assist in improving access to research tools (see Box 7-8). In practice, however, the exercise of some options may

BOX 7-8   Legal Authorities of NIH in Setting Intellectual Property Policy

Intramural Authorities

NIH has authority[1] to determine the patent, license, publication, and distribution policies that apply to the tools developed by NIH intramural scientists. In general, NIH does not file patent applications on technologies that are useful primarily as research tools and maintains a nonexclusive licensing policy for patented technologies that might be used as research tools. Further, when it enters into exclusive commercialization licenses, NIH reserves continuing rights over research uses, and when it grants exclusive license options on future discoveries, it seeks to ensure that the options do not attach to technologies useful primarily as research tools.

As a user of research tools generated by others, NIH can determine the terms it will accept in entering into license agreements and material transfer agreements (MTAs). As a matter of policy, NIH generally avoids giving an advance promise of future commercialization rights as a condition for obtaining a research tool.

Grants Authorities

As a funding agency charged with monitoring the use of grant funds and ensuring that the purposes of grants are carried out, NIH can set terms and conditions on grants and promulgate grant policies within the constraints of the Bayh-Dole Act. However, the policies currently in place apply piecemeal to isolated circumstances and have to date not been integrated into a single, cohesive policy directive.

Exceptional Circumstances of the Bayh-Dole Act

The Bayh-Dole Act gives NIH authority to establish funding agreement terms that limit the recipient's right to elect title, or to retain title itself, to inventions "in exceptional circumstances when it is determined by the agency that restriction or elimination of the right to retain title to any invention will better promote the objectives" of the law. NIH can use this authority if the primary purpose of the grant is to generate specific research tools, or an entire class of tools, that are likely to be widely disseminated and utilized if left in the public domain. As owner of these inventions, NIH can then decide for itself what patenting and licensing strategies make the most sense to ensure continuing availability of particular tools for further research, as well as to ensure incentives for commercialization. The difficulty with this approach is that it requires an ability to distinguish research tools from other discoveries. Moreover, some research tools may require the sort of private investment that is unlikely in the absence of an exclusive license before they will be developed to the point of achieving practical utilization. A less extreme step for NIH to take would be to delineate the circumstances under which the recipient could request greater rights, for example, if the recipient agreed to ensure the continuing availability of the research tool.

---

[1]This authority arises under the Bayh-Dole Act, 35 U.S.C. §§ 200-211, and Steven-Wydler Technology Innovation Act of 1980, 15 U.S.C. §§ 3701 et seq., as amended.

BOX 7-8 *continued*

Government Use License Stipulated by the Bayh-Dole Act

For all inventions developed in the course of NIH-funded research, the Bayh-Dole Act retains "a non-exclusive, nontransferable, irrevocable, paid-up license to practice or have practiced for or on behalf of the United States any subject invention throughout the world."[2] This license gives NIH, and any other agency of the federal government, the right to use any patented research tool arising in the course of federally sponsored research without liability for patent infringement. In practice, however, this license has not generally been used by NIH to obtain research tools from its grantees, either for its own intramural scientists or for dissemination to others. It is not clear whether NIH's retained license allows NIH to authorize use of inventions by other recipients of NIH grants. Some agencies take the position that the activities of grantees are covered by the exemption, but NIH has considered this an open question.

March-in Authority of the Bayh-Dole Act

The Bayh-Dole Act also has a mandatory licensing provision commonly referred to as the "march-in" authority.[3] The purpose of this provision is to prevent the underutilization of federally funded inventions. Prior to exercising march-in rights, the agency must determine that such action is necessary because of the failure of the contractor or its licensees to take effective steps to achieve practical application of the inventions in a particular field of use, to satisfy health or safety needs, or to meet requirements for public use specified by federal regulations. In contrast with the government use license, under the march-in provision, a third-party licensee could manufacture a tool and make it available for sale to the research community at large. The march-in authority has never been used. Although NIH was petitioned to use the authority in one instance, it elected not to use its authority to influence the marketplace (reviewed by Bar-Shalom and Cook-Deegan, 2002).

Rights of Government Agencies

Because of its status as an agency of the federal government, NIH has the authority to limit patent infringement against the government under 28 U.S.C. §1498. This statute gives the federal government the right to use and manufacture any patented invention without a license, but subject to liability for money damages, whether or not the invention was developed with federal funding. However, the exercise of this authority entails significant costs. The most obvious is the requirement that the government pay "reasonable and entire compensation," which could be a staggering amount if NIH were to exercise its rights on behalf of all its grantees and contractors. This authority also has the potential to undermine the value of patents in the hands of private owners.

---

[2]35 U.S.C. 202(c)(4).
[3]35 U.S.C. 203(1).
SOURCE: *Report of the NIH Working Group on Research Tools,* Appendix D (see <http://www.nih.gov/news/researchtools/appendd.htm>).

be perceived as extreme, and may have far-reaching and perhaps unpredictable consequences.

Providing funding to cover the costs of sharing materials could perhaps also facilitate a greater willingness to provide requested materials to fellow academic scientists (National Research Council, 2003).

Ultimately, assessing the impact of the increased assertion of intellectual property rights in academia due to the Bayh-Dole Act is difficult because few data that could be used for this purpose are reported back (Bar-Shalom and Cook-Deegan, 2002). A report of the U.S. Department of Health and Human Services (DHHS) (1994) notes many deficiencies in NIH's capability for monitoring patents that result from NIH funding. Consequently, NIH established a database to monitor invention disclosures and patents. Nonetheless, the General Accounting Office and the DHHS inspector general have since documented that NIH and other funding agencies still are not being notified of many patented inventions developed with federal funding (U.S. General Accounting Office, 1999). The General Accounting Office is currently conducting an investigation of the administration, use, and benefits to federal agencies of intellectual property derived from federally sponsored research (Aker, 2002). The President's Council of Advisors on Science and Technology has also been charged with assessing the benefits and difficulties of the Bayh-Dole Act with regard to the commercialization of products resulting from federally funded research, as well as with providing a review of technology transfer mechanisms. After collecting data and soliciting input from various stakeholders, such as small businesses and venture capital groups, the council plans to present the Bush Administration with its technology transfer recommendations in March 2003. Suggestions for major modifications to the act are not expected, however (Jenkins, 2002a, 2003a).

SUMMARY

Concerns have been raised in recent years about the willingness and ability of scientists and their institutions to share data, reagents, and other tools derived from their research. Many factors contribute to these difficulties, including the time and expense of sharing data and materials, the desire to protect raw or unpublished data and intellectual property, the incentive to maintain a lead in a particular research area, and the need to protect patient confidentiality. Since a primary goal of many large-scale biomedical research projects is to produce data and research tools these issues are of great importance when planning and conducting such projects. NIH should facilitate the sharing of data and the distribution of reagents to the extent feasible, by providing funds for the maintenance and distribution of reagents produced through large-scale projects, and by promoting broad dissemination of data and research tools generated with federal funds.

Over the course of the last two decades, the assignment and use of intellectual property rights have become increasingly common in the biomedical sciences. This phenomenon is due largely to changes in federal policy and legislation aimed at promoting the commercial development of discoveries made with public funding. There is evidence to suggest that biomedical patents assigned to academic research institutions are indeed generating research funds for those institutions and spawning research activities in the private sector. However, many questions have been raised regarding the licensing practices used by institutions to transfer their technologies to other institutions, both public and private. A number of licensing strategies exists for technology transfer, and the strategy chosen could greatly impact the accessibility of new discoveries to the scientific community. Unfortunately, however, little effort has been devoted to studying the impact of licensing practices on the use of patented biomedical innovations and on the progress of scientific research.

Patents and licensing practices have perhaps been most contentious for innovations that can be used as research tools for further research. Even a basic research project may require the use of several patented research tools, so it can be difficult, expensive, and time-consuming to acquire licenses for conducting such a project. Because the goal of many large-scale projects is to produce data and reagents that can be used as research tools, this issue may be especially salient for large-scale endeavors. NIH has many tools at its disposal to encourage and facilitate easy access to tools and discoveries derived from federally funded research. However, a lack of information on and scholarly assessment of licensing and technology transfer practices may be hindering effective action on the part of NIH. Thus, a systematic examination of the ways in which licensing practices affect the availability of research tools produced by and used for large-scale research projects could be extremely useful in formulating future NIH policies and actions.

8

Findings and Recommendations

The nature of biomedical research has been evolving in recent years. Relatively small projects initiated by single investigators have traditionally been and continue to be the mainstay of cancer research, as well as biomedical research in other fields. Recently, however, technological advances that make it easier to study the vast complexity of biological systems have led to the initiation of projects with a larger scale and scope. For instance, a new approach to biological experimentation known as "discovery science" first aims to develop a detailed inventory of genes, proteins, and metabolites in a particular cell type or tissue as a key information source (Lake and Hood, 2001). But even that information is not sufficient to understand the cell's complexity, so the ultimate goal of such research is to identify and characterize the elaborate networks of gene and protein interactions in the entire system that contribute to disease. This concept of systems biology is based on the premise that a disease can be fully comprehended only when its cause is understood from the molecular to the organismal level (Thomas and Gilbert, 2002). For example, rather than focusing on single aberrant genes or pathways, it is essential to understand the comprehensive and complex nature of cancer cells and their interaction with surrounding tissues. In many cases, large-scale analyses in which many parameters can be studied at once may be the most efficient and effective way to extract functional information and interactions from such complex biological systems.

The Human Genome Project is the biggest and best-known large-scale biomedical research project undertaken to date. Another project of that size is not likely to be launched in the near future, but many other projects that fall somewhere between the Human Genome Project and the traditional small projects have already been initiated, and many more have been contemplated. Indeed, the director of the National Institutes of Health (NIH) recently presented to his advisory council a "road map"[1] for the agency's future that includes a greater emphasis on "revolutionary methods of research" focused on scientific questions too complex to be addressed by the single-investigator scientific approach. He noted that the NIH grant process will need to be adapted to accommodate this new large-scale approach to scientific investigation, which may conflict with traditional paradigms for proposing, funding, and managing science projects that were designed for smaller-scale, hypothesis-driven research (Science and Government Alert, 2002).

Although the initial intent of this study was to examine large-scale cancer research, it quickly became clear that issues pertaining to large-scale science projects have broad implications that cut across all sectors and fields of biomedical research. Large-scale endeavors in the biomedical sciences often involve multiple disciplines and contribute to many fields and specialties. The Human Genome Project is a classic example of this concept, in that its products can benefit all fields of biology and biomedicine. The same is likely to be true for many other large-scale projects now under consideration or underway, such as the Protein Structure Initiative (PSI) and the International HapMap Project. Furthermore, given the funding structures of NIH, the launch of a large-scale project in one field could potentially impact progress as well as funding in other fields. Thus, while this report emphasizes examples from cancer research whenever feasible, the committee's recommendations are generally not specific to the National Cancer Institute (NCI) or to the field of cancer research; rather, they are directed toward the biomedical research community as a whole. Indeed, it is the committee's belief that all fields of biomedical research, including cancer research, could benefit from implementation of the recommendations presented herein.

Ideally, large-scale and small-scale research should complement each other and work synergistically to advance the field of biomedical research in the long term. For example, many large-scale projects generate hypotheses that can then be tested in smaller research projects. However, the new large-scale research opportunities are challenging traditional academic research structures because the projects are bigger, more costly,

---

[1]More than 100 scientists were consulted during the plan's preparation, and all of the agency's Institute and Center directors discussed it during a two-day retreat held in September 2002. Additional consultations are now planned with extramural researchers, as well as public and patient groups.

often more technologically sophisticated, and require greater planning and oversight. These challenges raise the question of how the large-scale approach to biomedical research could be improved if such projects are to be undertaken in the future.

Ideally, large-scale and small-scale research should complement each other and work synergistically to advance the field of biomedical research in the long term. For example, many large-scale projects generate hypotheses that can then be tested in smaller research projects. However, the new large-scale research opportunities are challenging traditional academic research structures because the projects are bigger, more costly, often more technologically sophisticated, and require greater planning and oversight. These challenges raise the question of how the large-scale approach to biomedical research could be improved if such projects are to be undertaken in the future. The committee concluded[2] that such improvement could be achieved by adopting the seven recommendations presented here to address these issues.

The first three recommendations suggest a number of changes in the way scientific opportunities for large-scale research are initially assessed as they emerge from the scientific community, as well as in the way specific projects are subsequently selected, funded, launched, and evaluated. Although the procedures of NIH and other federal agencies have a degree of flexibility that has allowed some large-scale research endeavors to be undertaken, a mechanism is needed through which input from innovators in research can be routinely collected and incorporated into the institutional decision-making processes. Also needed is a more standard mechanism for vetting various proposals for large-scale projects. For example, none of the large projects initiated by NCI to date has been evaluated in a systematic manner. There is also a need for greater planning and oversight by federal sponsors during both the initiation and phase-out of a large-scale project. Careful assessment of past and current large-scale projects to identify best practices and determine whether the large-scale approach adds value to the traditional models of research would also provide highly useful information for future endeavors.

Recommendation 1: NIH and other federal funding agencies that support large-scale biomedical science (including the National Science Foundation [NSF], the U.S. Department of Energy [DOE], the

---

[2] The findings and recommendations presented in this chapter are based on the information reviewed in the previous chapters, which include literature reviews, compilations of data, and summaries of findings. Detailed discussions and references can be found in those chapters and are merely summarized here.

U.S. Department of Agriculture [USDA], and the U.S. Department of Defense [DOD]) should develop a more open and systematic method for assessing important new research opportunities emerging from the scientific community in which a large-scale approach is likely to achieve the scientific goals more effectively or efficiently than traditional research efforts.

- This method should include a mechanism for soliciting and evaluating proposals from individuals or small groups as well as from large groups, but in either case, broad consultation within the relevant scientific community should occur before funding is made available, perhaps through ad hoc public conferences. Whenever feasible, these discussions should be NIH-wide and multidisciplinary.
- An NIH-wide, transinstitute panel of experts appointed by the NIH director would facilitate the vetting process for assessing scientific opportunities that could benefit from a large-scale approach.
- Once the most promising concepts for large-scale research have been selected by the director's panel, appropriate guidelines for peer review of specific project proposals should be established. These guidelines should be applied by the institutions that oversee the projects.
- Collaborations among institutes could encourage participation by smaller institutes that may not have the resources to launch their own large-scale projects.
- NIH should continue to explore alternative funding mechanisms for large-scale endeavors, perhaps including approaches similar to those used by NCI's Unconventional Innovations Program, as well as funding collaborations with industry and other federal funding agencies.
- International collaborations should be encouraged, but an approach for achieving such cooperation should be determined on a case by case basis.

Recommendation 2: Large-scale research endeavors should have clear but flexible plans for entry into and phase out from projects once the stated ends have been achieved.

- It is essential to define the goals of a project clearly and to monitor and assess its progress regularly against well-defined milestones.
- Carefully planning and orchestrating the launch of a large-scale project is imperative for its long-term success and efficiency.
- NIH should be very cautious about establishing permanent infrastructures, such as centers or institutes, to undertake large-scale projects, in order to avoid the accumulation of additional Institutes via this mechanism.

- Historically, NIH has not had a good mechanism for phasing out established research programs, but large-scale projects should not become institutionalized by default simply because of their size.
- If national centers with short-term missions are to be established, this should be done with a clear understanding that they are temporary and are not meant to continue once a project has been completed.
  - Leasing space is one way to facilitate downsizing upon completion of a project.
  - Phase-out funding could enable investigators to downsize over a period of 2–3 years.

Recommendation 3: NCI and NIH, as well as other federal funding agencies that support large-scale biomedical science, should commission a thorough analysis of their recent large-scale initiatives once they are well established to determine whether those efforts have been effective and efficient in achieving their stated goals and to aid in the planning of future large-scale projects.

- NIH should develop a set of metrics for assessing the technical and scientific output (such as data and research tools) of large-scale projects. The assessment should include an evaluation of whether the field has benefited from such a project in terms of increased speed of discoveries and their application or a reduction in costs.
- The assessment should be undertaken by external, independent peer review panels with relevant expertise that include academic, government, and industry scientists.
- To help guide future large-scale projects, the assessment should pay particular attention to a project's management and organizational structure, including how scientific and program managers and staff were selected, trained, and retained and how well they performed.
- The assessment should include tracking of any trainees involved in a project (graduate students and postdoctoral scientists) to determine the value of the training environment and the impact on career trajectories.
- The assessment should examine the impact of industry contracts or collaborations within large-scale research projects. Industry has many potential strengths to offer such projects, including efficiency and effective project management and staffing, but intellectual property issues represent a potential barrier to such collaborations. Thus, some balance must be sought between providing incentives for producing the data and facilitating the research community's access to the resultant data.

– In pursuing large-scale projects with industry, NIH should carefully consider the data dissemination goals of the endeavor before making the funds available.

– To the extent appropriate, NIH should mandate timely and unrestricted release of data within the terms of the grant or contract, in the same spirit as the Bermuda rules adopted for the release of data in the Human Genome Project.

The committee has formulated four additional recommendations aimed at improving the conduct of possible future large-scale projects. These recommendations emerged from the committee's identification of various potential obstacles to conducting a large-scale research project successfully and efficiently. To begin with, human resources are key to the success of any large-scale project. If large-scale projects are deemed worthy of substantial sums of federal support, they also clearly warrant the highest-caliber staff to perform and oversee the work. But if qualified individuals, especially at the doctoral level, are expected to participate in such undertakings, they must have sufficient incentives to take on the risks and responsibilities involved. In particular, effective administrative management and committed scientific leadership are crucial for meeting expected milestones on schedule and within budget; thus the success of a large-scale project is greatly dependent upon the skills and knowledge of the scientists and administrators who manage it, including those within the federal funding agencies. However, it may be quite difficult to recruit staff with the skills to meet this need because of the unusual status of such managerial positions within the scientific career structure, and because scientists rarely undergo formal training in management. Young investigators and trainees also need recognition for their efforts that contribute to elaborate, long-term, and large multi-institutional efforts. Thus, the committee concluded that both universities and government agencies need to develop new approaches for assessing teamwork and management, as well as novel ways of recognizing and rewarding accomplishment in such positions.

Recommendation 4: Institutions should develop the necessary incentives for recruiting and retaining qualified scientific managers and staff for large-scale projects, and for recognizing and rewarding scientific collaborations and team-building efforts.

• Funding agencies should develop appropriate career paths for individuals who serve as program managers for the large-scale projects they fund.

• Academic institutions should develop appropriate career paths, including suitable criteria for performance evaluation and promotion, for those individuals who manage and staff large-scale collaborative projects carried out under their purview.

- Industry and The National Laboratories may both serve as instructive models in achieving these goals, as they have a history of rewarding scientists for their participation in team-oriented research.
- It is important to establish guiding principles for such issues as equitable pay and benefits, job stability, and potential for advancement to avoid relegating these valuable scientists and managers to a "second-tier" status. Federal agencies should provide adequate funding to universities engaged in large-scale biomedical research projects so that these individuals can be sufficiently compensated for their role and contribution.
- Universities, especially those engaged in large-scale research, should develop training programs for scientists involved in such projects. Examples include courses dealing with such topics as managing teams of people and working toward milestones within timelines. Input from industry experts who deal routinely with these issues would be highly valuable.

The committee also identified potential impediments to deriving the greatest benefits from the products of large-scale endeavors in terms of scientific progress for biomedical research in general. Large-scale projects are most likely to speed the progress of biomedical research as a whole when their products are made widely available to the broad scientific community. However, concerns have been raised in recent years about the willingness and ability of scientists and their institutions to share data, reagents, and other tools derived from their research. Since a primary goal of many large-scale biomedical research projects is to produce data and research tools, NIH should facilitate the sharing of data and the distribution of reagents to the extent feasible. Currently, NIH grants generally do not provide funds for this purpose, making it difficult for investigators to maintain reagents and share them with the research community. This obstacle could be reduced if NIH provided such funds for large-scale research projects.

Recommendation 5: NIH should draft contracts with industry to preserve reagents and other research tools and distribute them to the scientific community once they have been produced through large-scale projects.

- The Pathogen Functional Genomics Resource Center, established through a contract with the National Institute of Allergy and Infectious Diseases, could serve as a model for this undertaking.
- The distribution of standardized and quality-controlled reagents

and tools would improve the quality of the data obtained through research and make it easier to compare data from different investigators.

- Producing the reagents and making them widely available to many researchers would be more cost-effective than providing funds to a few scientists to produce their own.

An issue closely related to the sharing of data and reagents is the licensing of intellectual property. Many concerns have been raised in recent years about the challenges and expenses associated with the transfer of patented technology from one organization to another. Innovations that can be used as research tools may offer the greatest challenge in this regard because it is difficult to predict the future applications and value of a particular tool, and because a number of different tools may be needed for a single research project. Since many large-scale projects in the biosciences aim to produce data and other tools for future research, this subject is especially salient for large-scale research. The committee concluded that NIH should continue to promote the broad accessibility of research tools derived from federally funded large-scale research to the extent feasible, while at the same time considering the appropriate role for intellectual property rights in a given project. However, in the absence of adequate information and scholarly assessment, it is difficult to determine how NIH could best accomplish that goal. Thus, the committee recommends that such an assessment be undertaken, and that appropriate actions be taken based on the findings of the study.

Recommendation 6: NIH should commission a study to examine systematically the ways in which licensing practices affect the availability of research tools produced by and used for large-scale biomedical research projects.

- Whenever possible, NIH and NCI should use their leverage and resources to promote the free and open exchange of scientific knowledge and information, and to help minimize the time and expense of technology transfer.
- Depending on the findings of the proposed study, NIH should promote licensing practices that facilitate broad access to research tools by issuing licensing guidelines for NIH-funded discoveries.

In addition to the role of federal funding agencies, the committee considered the role of industry and philanthropies in conducting large-scale biomedical research. Public–private collaborations provide a way to share the costs and risks of innovative research, as well as the benefits. Philanthropies and other nonprofit organizations can play an important role in launching nontraditional projects that do not fit well with federal funding mechanisms. Pharmaceutical and biotechnology companies also make enormous contributions to biomedical research worldwide. Traditionally, the role of independent companies has been to pursue applied research aimed at producing an end product; however, the distinction between "applied" and "basic" research has blurred in recent years, in part because of novel approaches used for drug discovery and development. A recent focus by academic scientists on translational research, which aims to translate fundamental discoveries into clinically useful practices, has further obscured the distinction.

Several recent projects initiated and funded by industry or carried out in cooperation with industry and nonprofit organizations clearly demonstrate the potential value of contributions by these entities to large-scale research endeavors. The Single Nucleotide Polymorphism, or SNP, Consortium is a prime example of how effective these sectors can be when involved in a large-scale research projects. Industry in particular has many inherent strengths that could be brought to bear on large-scale biomedical research efforts, such as experience in coordinating and managing teams of scientists working toward a common goal. Combining the respective strengths of academia and industry could optimize the pace of biomedical research and development, potentially leading to more rapid improvements in human health. Thus, the committee recommends that cooperation between academia and industry be encouraged for large-scale research projects whenever feasible.

> **Recommendation 7: Given the changing nature of biomedical research, consideration should be given to pursuing projects initiated by academic scientists in cooperation with industry to achieve the goals of large-scale research. When feasible, such cooperative efforts could entail collaborative projects, as well as direct funding of academic research by industry, if the goals of the research are mutually beneficial.**

- Academia is generally best suited for making scientific discoveries, while the strength of industry most often lies in its ability to develop or add value to these discoveries.
- Establishing a more seamless connection between the two endeavors could greatly facilitate translational research and thus speed clinical applications of new discoveries.

Great strides in biomedical research have been made in recent decades, due largely to a robust investigator-initiated research enterprise. Recent technological advances have provided new opportunities to further accelerate the pace of discovery through large-scale research initiatives that can provide valuable information and tools to facilitate this traditional approach to experimentation. Recent large-scale collaborations have also allowed scientists to tackle complex research questions that could not readily be addressed by a single investigator or institution. The current leadership of NIH and many scientists in the field clearly have expressed an interest in integrating the discovery approach to biomedical science with hypothesis-driven experimentation. As a result, at least some large-scale endeavors in the biomedical sciences are likely to be undertaken in the future as well. But because the large-scale approach is relatively new to the life sciences, there are few precedents to follow or learn from when planning and launching a new large-scale project. Moreover, there has been little formal or scholarly assessment of large-scale projects already undertaken.

Now is the time to address the critical issues identified in this report in order to optimize future investments in large-scale endeavors, whatever they may be. The ultimate goal of biomedical research, both large- and small-scale, is to advance knowledge and provide society with useful innovations. Determining the best and most efficient method for accomplishing that goal, however, is a continuing and evolving challenge. Following the recommendations presented here could facilitate a move toward a more open, inclusive, and accountable approach to large-scale biomedical research, and help strike the appropriate balance between large- and small-scale research to maximize progress in understanding and controlling human disease.

References

ABT Associates, Inc. 1996. An Evaluation of the NSF Science and Technology Centers (STC) Program. Cambridge, MA: Center for Science and Technology Policy Studies.

AIP Center for History of Physics. 1992. AIP Study of Multi-Institutional Collaborations. Phase I: High-Energy Physics. Report Number 1: Summary of Project and Findings: Project Recommendations. College Park, MD: American Institute of Physics.

Abbott A. 2001. Workshop prepares ground for human proteome project. *Nature* 413(6858): 763.

Adam D. 2001a. Database of molecular probes set to boost chemical genetics. *Nature* 411(6840):873.

Adam D. 2001b. Genetics group targets disease markers in the human sequence. *Nature* 412(6843):105.

Aker J. 2002. Access to intellectual property under Bayh/Dole subject of Markey GAO investigation request. Washington, DC: Washington Fax.

Alper J. 1999. From the bioweapons trenches, new tools for battling microbes. *Science* 284(5421):1754–5.

Anderson PW. 1999. Why do they leave physics? *Physics Today* 52(9): 11.

Austin R. 2002. Project management and discovery. *Science* Next Wave September 13. See <http://nextwave.sciencemag.org>.

Bar-Shalom A, Cook-Deegan R. 2002. Patents and innovations in cancer therapeutics: Lessons from cell pro. *The Millbank Quarterly* 80(4).

Barinaga M. 2000. Scientific community. Soft money's hard realities. *Science* 289(5487):2024–8.

Blumenthal D, Campbell EG, Anderson MS, Causino N, Louis KS. 1997. Withholding research results in academic life science. Evidence from a national survey of faculty. JAMA 277(15):1224-8.

Boahene AK. 2002. Patented genetic sequences would be available to researchers under Rivers bill. Washington, DC: Washington Fax.

Brunak S, Danchin A, Hattori M, Nakamura H, Shinozaki K, Matise T, Preuss D. 2002. Nucleotide sequence database policies. *Science* 298(5597):1333.

Burley SK. 2000. An overview of structural genomics. *Nat Struct Biol* 7 Suppl:932–4.

Campbell EG, Clarridge BR, Gokhale M, Birenbaum L, Hilgartner S, Holtzman NA, Blumenthal D. 2002. Data withholding in academic genetics: evidence from a national survey. JAMA 287:473–80.

Cancer Letter. 2001. *NCI, NIGMS To Support Synchotron Beamlines.* The Cancer Letter 27(42) November 16. Washington, DC: Cancer Letter Publicatons.

Check E. 2002. NIH ponders issues of scale in protein push. *Nature* 417(6885):107.

Chicurel M. 2001. Faster, better, cheaper genotyping. *Nature* 412(6847):580–2.

Clarke J, Piccolo J, Stanton B, Tyson K. 2000. Patent Pools: A Solution to the Problem of Access in Biotechnology Patents. Washington, DC: United States Patent and Trademark Office.

Cohen J. 1999. Philanthropy's rising tide lifts science. *Science* 286(5438):214–23.

Cohen J. 2002. Public health. Gates Foundation rearranges public health universe. *Science* 295(5562):2000.

Cook-Deegan RM. 1994. The Gene Wars: Science, Politics, and the Human Genome. New York: W.W. Norton & Company.

Couzin J. 2002a. Genomics. New mapping project splits the community. *Science* 296(5572): 1391–3.

Couzin J. 2002b. Human genome. HapMap launched with pledges of $100 million. *Science* 298(5595):941–2.

Couzin J, Enserink M. 2002. Women's health. More questions about hormone replacement. *Science* 298(5595):942.

Crow M, Bozeman B. 2001. Limited By Design: R&D Laboratories in the U.S. National Innovation System. New York: Columbia University Press.

Culliton B. 1974. Virus cancer program: Review panel stands by criticism. *Science* 184(4133): 143–5.

Davies K. 2001. Cracking the Genome: Inside the Race to Unlock Human DNA. New York: Free Press.

Davis BD. 1990. The human genome and other initiatives. *Science* 249(4967):342–3.

Davis M. 2000. Sorting basic research into disease categories is a nightmare for NIH administrators, yet patient advocates, many in Congress, think in those terms. Washington, DC: Washington Fax.

DeVita VT, Goldin A. 1984. Therapeutic research in the National Cancer Institute. NIH: An account of research in its laboratories and clinics. Orlando, FL: Academic Press.

Ducor P. 1997. Are patents and research compatible? *Nature* 387(6628):13–4.

Dulbecco R. 1986. A turning point in cancer research: sequencing the human genome. *Science* 231(4742):1055–6.

Edwards M. 1996. 360 Feedback: The Powerful New Model for Employee Assessment and Performance Improvement. New York: Amacom Books.

Eisenberg RS. 1997. Chapter 2. National Research Council. Intellectual Property Rights and the Dissemination of Research Tools in Molecular Biology. Washington, DC: National Academy Press.

Eisenberg RS. 2000. Genomics in the public domain: strategy and policy. *Nat Rev Genet* 1(1):70–4.

Encyclopedia Brittanica. 2003. See <http://www.britannica.com>.

Enserink M. 2002a. Epidemiology. Despite safety concerns, U.K. hormone study to proceed. *Science* 297(5581):492.

Enserink M. 2002b. Women's health. The vanishing promises of hormone replacement. *Science* 297(5580):325–6.

Ergenzinger E, Spruill M. 2003. Basic science in U.S. universities can infringe patents. *The Scientist* 17(5):43.

Freeman R, Weinstein E, Marincola E, Rosenbaum J, Solomon F. 2001. Careers. Competition and careers in biosciences. *Science* 294(5550):2293–4.

Funding First Collection. 2000. Exceptional Returns: The Economic Value of America's Investment in Medical Research. New York: Funding First.

Galison P, Hevly B, 1992. Big Science: The Growth of Large-Scale Research. Stanford: Stanford University Press.

Gallo RC. 1999. Thematic review series. XI: Viruses in the origin of human cancer. Introduction and overview. *Proc Assoc Am Physicians* 111:560–2.

Gallo RC, Mann D, Broder S, Ruscetti FW, Maeda M, Kalyanaraman VS, Robert-Guroff M, Reitz MS Jr. 1982. Human T-cell leukemia-lymphoma virus (HTLV) is in T but not B lymphocytes from a patient with cutaneous T-cell lymphoma. *Proc Natl Acad Sci U S A* 79:5680–3.

Gershon D. 2000. Vaccine centres unite specialists in the battle against infectious diseases. *Nature* 408(6813):753–4.

Gillespie G, Chubin D, Kurzon G. 1985. Experience with the NIH peer review: researcher's cynicism and desire for change. *Science, Technology, and Human Value* 10:44–53.

Glanz J. 1998. Careers: Young physicists despair of tenured jobs. *Science* 279(5354):1128.

Golde CM, Dore, TM. 2001. At Cross Purposes: What the Experiences of Doctoral Students Reveal about Doctoral Education (<www.phd-survey.org>). Philadelphia, PA: A report prepared for The Pew Charitable Trusts.

Goldberg S. 1995. Big Science: Atomic Bomb Research and the Beginnings of High Energy Physics. Seattle: History of Science Society.

Goldman E, Marshall E. 2002. Research funding. NIH grantees: where have all the young ones gone? *Science* 298(5591):40–1.

Green W. 1995. Two Cheers for Democracy: Science and Technology Politics. New York: Center for Science, Policy, and Outcomes.

Greenberg DS. 2001. Science, Money, and Politics: Political Triumph and Ethical Erosion. Chicago: University of Chicago Press.

Gross CP, Anderson GF, Powe NR. 1999. The relation between funding by the National Institutes of Health and the burden of disease. *N Engl J Med* 340:1881–7.

Hackett E. 1987. The plight of academic "marginals". *The Scientist* 1(18):13.

Hafner L. 2001. Rat genome project shifts to whole-genome shotgun, adds pioneer Celera. Washington, DC: Washington Fax.

Hafner L. 2002. Rigorous OMB performance measures will be used to frame agency budget proposals for FY 2004. Washington, DC: Washington Fax.

Haley S. 2000. The public and most of Congress believe there is a direct relationship between investment and cure, warns AAAS fellow. Washington, DC: Washington Fax.

Haley S. 2001. Kirschstein tells how NIH is adapting to the evolving multidisciplinary research model. Washington, DC: Washington Fax.

Haywood HL. 1923. Freemasonry and the Guild System. *The Builder*.

Heilbron JL, Kevles DJ. 1988. Finding a policy for mapping and sequencing the human genome: Lessons from the history of particle physics. *Minerva* 26:299–314.

Heinig SJ, Quon AS, Meyer RE, Korn D. 1999. The changing landscape for clinical research. *Acad Med* 74:726–45.

Heller MA, Eisenberg RS. 1998. Can patents deter innovation? The anticommons in biomedical research. *Science* 280(5364):698–701.

Helmuth L. 2001. Genome research: map of the human genome 3.0. *Science* 293(5530):583–5.

Hendler J. 2003. Communication. Science and the semantic web. *Science* 299(5606):520–1.

Henry MR, Cho MK, Weaver MA, Merz JF. 2002. Genetics. DNA patenting and licensing. *Science* 297(5585):1279.

Institute of Medicine. 1994. Careers in Clinical Research: Obstacles and Opportunities. Washington, DC: National Academy Press.

Institute of Medicine. 1996. Resource Sharing in Biomedical Research. Washington, DC: National Academy Press.

Institute of Medicine. 1998. Scientific Opportunities and Public Needs: Improving Priority Setting and Public Input at the National Institutes of Health. Washington, DC: National Academy Press.

Institute of Medicine. 2000. Summary of the June 2000 Meeting of the Clinical Research Round Table. Washington, DC: National Academy Press.

Jenkins SC. 2002a. PCAST Bayh-Dole assessment likely will address investment recovery. Washington, DC: Washington Fax.

Jenkins SC. 2002b. Proactively shaping control arrangements can ensure data access, Duke's Reichman tells science community. Washington, DC: Washington Fax.

Jenkins SC. 2003a. President's science and technology council to advise administration on tech transfer policy in March. Washington, DC: Washington Fax.

Jenkins SC. 2003b. Two percent NIH FY 2000 budget increase would reduce new grants by 1000 FASEB says. Washington, DC: Washington Fax.

Kaiser J. 2001. Bioinformatics. Hughes to build own tech research center. *Science* 291(5505): 803.

Kaiser J. 2002. Proteomics. Public-private group maps out initiatives. *Science* 296(5569):827.

Kevles DJ, Hood L. 1992. The Code of Codes: Scientific and Social Issues in the Human Genome Project. Cambridge, MA: Harvard University Press.

Korn D, Rich RR, Garrison HH, Golub SH, Hendrix MJ, Heinig SJ, Masters BS, Turman RJ. 2002. Science policy. The NIH budget in the "postdoubling" era. *Science* 296(5572):1401–2.

Kyd J. 2000. New PTO guidelines released. Added utility requirement may cause problems for biomedical researchers. Washington, DC: Washington Fax.

Lake G, Hood LE. 2001. Big computing comes to biology. *Nature Yearbook of Science and Technology*. Washington, DC: Nature Publishing Group: 82–5.

Lander ES, Linton LM, Birren B, Nusbaum C, Zody MC, Baldwin J, Devon K, Dewar K, Doyle M, FitzHugh W, Funke R, Gage D, Harris K, Heaford A, Howland J, Kann L, Lehoczky J, LeVine R, McEwan P, McKernan K, Meldrim J, Mesirov JP, Miranda C, Morris W, Naylor J, Raymond C, Rosetti M, Santos R, Sheridan A, Sougnez C, Stange-Thomann N, Stojanovic N, Subramanian A, Wyman D, Rogers J, Sulston J, Ainscough R, Beck S, Bentley D, Burton J, Clee C, Carter N, Coulson A, Deadman R, Deloukas P, Dunham A, Dunham I, Durbin R, French L, Grafham D, Gregory S, Hubbard T, Humphray S, Hunt A, Jones M, Lloyd C, McMurray A, Matthews L, Mercer S, Milne S, Mullikin JC, Mungall A, Plumb R, Ross M, Shownkeen R, Sims S, Waterston RH, Wilson RK, Hillier LW, McPherson JD, Marra MA, Mardis ER, Fulton LA, Chinwalla AT, Pepin KH, Gish WR, Chissoe SL, Wendl MC, Delehaunty KD, Miner TL, Delehaunty A, Kramer JB, Cook LL, Fulton RS, Johnson DL, Minx PJ, Clifton SW, Hawkins T, Branscomb E, Predki P, Richardson P, Wenning S, Slezak T, Doggett N, Cheng JF, Olsen A, Lucas S, Elkin C, Uberbacher E, Frazier M, Gibbs RA, Muzny DM, Scherer SE, Bouck JB, Sodergren EJ, Worley KC, Rives CM, Gorrell JH, Metzker ML, Naylor SL, Kucherlapati RS, Nelson DL, Weinstock GM, Sakaki Y, Fujiyama A, Hattori M, Yada T, Toyoda A, Itoh T, Kawagoe C, Watanabe H, Totoki Y, Taylor T, Weissenbach J, Heilig R, Saurin W, Artiguenave F, Brottier P, Bruls T, Pelletier E, Robert C, Wincker P, Smith DR, Doucette-Stamm L, Rubenfield M, Weinstock K, Lee HM, Dubois J, Rosenthal A, Platzer M, Nyakatura G, Taudien S, Rump A, Yang H, Yu J, Wang J, Huang G, Gu J, Hood L, Rowen L, Madan A, Qin S, Davis RW, Federspiel NA, Abola AP, Proctor MJ, Myers RM, Schmutz J, Dickson M, Grimwood J, Cox DR, Olson MV,

Kaul R, Raymond C, Shimizu N, Kawasaki K, Minoshima S, Evans GA, Athanasiou M, Schultz R, Roe BA, Chen F, Pan H, Ramser J, Lehrach H, Reinhardt R, McCombie WR, de la Bastide M, Dedhia N, Blocker H, Hornischer K, Nordsiek G, Agarwala R, Aravind L, Bailey JA, Bateman A, Batzoglou S, Birney E, Bork P, Brown DG, Burge CB, Cerutti L, Chen HC, Church D, Clamp M, Copley RR, Doerks T, Eddy SR, Eichler EE, Furey TS, Galagan J, Gilbert JG, Harmon C, Hayashizaki Y, Haussler D, Hermjakob H, Hokamp K, Jang W, Johnson LS, Jones TA, Kasif S, Kaspryzk A, Kennedy S, Kent WJ, Kitts P, Koonin EV, Korf I, Kulp D, Lancet D, Lowe TM, McLysaght A, Mikkelsen T, Moran JV, Mulder N, Pollara VJ, Ponting CP, Schuler G, Schultz J, Slater G, Smit AF, Stupka E, Szustakowski J, Thierry-Mieg D, Thierry-Mieg J, Wagner L, Wallis J, Wheeler R, Williams A, Wolf YI, Wolfe KH, Yang SP, Yeh RF, Collins F, Guyer MS, Peterson J, Felsenfeld A, Wetterstrand KA, Patrinos A, Morgan MJ, Szustakowki J, de Jong P, Catanese JJ, Osoegawa K, Shizuya H, Choi S, Chen YJ. 2001. Initial sequencing and analysis of the human genome. *Nature* 409(6822):860–921.

Lawler A. 2003. University-industry collaboration. Last of the big-time spenders? *Science* 299(5605):330–3.

Lazear EP, Rosen S. 1981. Rank order tournaments as optimal labor contracts. *J Polit Econ* 89:841–864.

Lekowski W. 1999. Research results can be measured for performance review, says COSEPUP. Even basic research can be measured according to certain standards. Washington, DC: Washington Fax.

Levin R, Klevorick A, Nelson R, Winter S. 1987. Appropriating the returns from industrial research and development. Brookings Papers on Economic Activity. Brookings Institute, Washington, DC: 783-832.

Lewis R. 2001. News—A personal view of genomics. *The Scientist* 15(23):10.

Loder N. 2000. Celera's shotgun approach puts *Drosophila* in the bag. *Nature* 403(6772): 817.

Longfellow D. 2000. Introductory Remarks. Estrogens As Endogenous Carcinogens in the Breast and Prostate. Conference Proceedings. Chantilly, Virginia, USA. March 15–17, 1998. Journal of the National Cancer Institute Monographs 27:13–5.

Macilwain C. 2000. World leaders heap praise on human genome landmark. *Nature* 405(6790): 983–5.

Malakoff D. 1999. Military research: Pentagon agency thrives on in-your-face science. *Science* 285(5433):1476–9.

Malakoff D. 2001. Functional genomics. Pathogen researchers get help from TIGR. *Science* 294(5549):2069–70.

Malakoff D. 2003. Intellectual property. Universities ask Supreme Court to reverse patent ruling. *Science* 299(5603):26–7.

Marshall E. 1997. Too radical for NIH? Try DARPA. *Science* 275(5301):744–6.

Marshall E. 1999. New NIH rules promote greater sharing of tools and materials. *Science* 286(5449):2430-1.

Marshall E. 2000. Genomics. Public-private project to deliver mouse genome in 6 months. *Science* 290(5490):242–3.

Marshall E. 2001. Genome sequencing. Celera assembles mouse genome; public labs plan new strategy. *Science* 292(5518):822.

Marshall E. 2002a. Intellectual property. DuPont ups ante on use of Harvard's OncoMouse. *Science* 296(5571):1212.

Marshall E. 2002b. Genome sequencing. Public group completes draft of the mouse. *Science* 296(5570):1005.

Marshall E. 2002c. Data sharing. DNA sequencer protests being scooped with his own data. *Science* 295(5558):1206-7.

Maurer SM, Hugenholtz PB, Onsrud HJ. 2001. Intellectual property. Europe's database experiment. *Science* 294(5543):789–90.

McGeary and Burstein. 1999. Sources of Cancer Research Funding in the United States. Washington, DC: Institute of Medicine.

McGeary and Merrill. 1999. Recent trends in federal spending on scientific and engineering research: Impacts on research fields and graduate training. (Appendix A). STEP Board. Securing America's Industrial Strength. Washington, DC: National Academy Press.

Mervis J. 2002. Research centers. Science with an agenda: NSF expands centers program. *Science* 297(5581):506–9.

Metheny B. 2002. NIH reorganization should be thematic, relevant to the public perception of medical research, panelists advise. Washington, DC: Washington Fax.

Nathan D. 1997. NIH Director's Panel on Clinical Research Report to the Advisory Committee to the NIH Director. Bethesda, MD: National Institutes of Health.

Nathanson KL, Shugart YY, Omaruddin R, Szabo C, Goldgar D, Rebbeck TR, Weber BL. 2002. CGH-targeted linkage analysis reveals a possible BRCA1 modifier locus on chromosome 5q. *Hum Mol Genet* 11:1327–32.

National Academy of Public Administration (NAPA). 1995. National Science Foundation's Science and Technology Centers: Building an Interdisciplinary Research Program. Washington, DC: NAPA.

National Academy of Sciences. 1999. Evaluating Federal Research Programs: Research and the Government Performance and Results Act. Washington, DC: National Academy Press.

National Academy of Sciences. 2001. Implementing the Government Performance and Results Act for Research: A Status Report. Washington, DC: National Academy Press.

National Cancer Advisory Board. 1974. Report of the Ad Hoc Review Committee of the Virus Cancer Program. Bethesda, MD: National Cancer Institute.

National Cancer Advisory Board: Ad Hoc Working Group on the NCI Intramural Research Program. 1995. A Review of the Intramural Program of the NCI (Bishop Calabresi Report). Bethesda, MD: National Cancer Institute.

National Cancer Advisory Board. Report of the P30/P50 Ad Hoc Working Group. 2003. Advancing Translational Cancer Research: A Vision of the Cancer Center and SPORE Programs of the Future. Bethesda, MD: National Cancer Institute.

National Institutes of Health. 1998. Report of the NIH Working Group on Research Tools. Bethesda, MD: National Institutes of Health.

National Research Council. 1988. Mapping and Sequencing the Human Genome. Washington, DC: National Academy Press.

National Research Council. 1994a. A Space Physics Paradox. Washington, DC: National Academy Press.

National Research Council. 1994b. Sharing Laboratory Resources: Genetically Altered Mice. Washington, DC: National Academy Press.

National Research Council, Committee on Criteria for Federal Support of Research and Development. 1995. Allocating Federal Funds for Science and Technology. Washington, DC: National Academy Press.

National Research Council, COSEPUP. 1996. An assessment of the National Science Foundation's Science and Technology Centers Program. Washington, DC: National Academy Press.

National Research Council. 1997. Intellectual Property Rights and the Dissemination of Research Tools in Molecular Biology. Washington, DC: National Academy Press.

National Research Council. 1998a. Trends in the Early Careers of Life Scientists. Washington, DC: National Academy Press.

National Research Council. 1998b. Serving Science and Society in the New Millenium. Washington, DC: National Academy Press.

National Research Council. 1999. A Question of Balance: Private Rights and the Public Interest in Scientific and Technical Databases. Washington, DC: National Academy Press.

National Research Council. 2000. Enhancing the Postdoctoral Experience for Scientists and Engineers. Washington, DC: National Academy Press.

National Research Council. 2001a. Trends in Federal Support of Research and Graduate Education. Washington DC: National Academy Press.

National Research Council. 2001b. Physics in a New Era. Washington, DC: National Academy Press.

National Research Council. 2003. Sharing Publication-Related Data and Materials: Responsibilities of Authorship in the Life Sciences. Washington, DC: The National Academies Press.

National Science Foundation. 2002. Science and Engineering Indicators—2002. Arlington, VA: National Science Foundation.

Norberg A, O'Neill JE. 1996. Transforming Computer Technology: Information Processing for the Pentagon, 1962–86. Baltimore: Johns Hopkins University Press.

Office of Technology Assessment. 1991. Federally Funded Research: Decisions for a Decade. Washington, DC: OTA.

Pennisi E. 1998. DNA sequencers' trial by fire. *Science* 280(5365):814–7.

Pennisi E. 1999. Fruitfly researchers sign pact with Celera. *Science* 283(5403):767.

Pennisi E. 2000a. Genomics. Fruit fly genome yields data and validation. *Science* 287(5457): 1374.

Pennisi E. 2000b. Genomics. Mouse sequencers take up the shotgun. *Science* 287(5456):1179, 1181.

Pennisi E. 2002a. Genomics. Genome centers push for polished draft. *Science* 296(5573): 1600–1.

Pennisi E. 2002b. Human genome project. Genome institute wrestles mightily with its future. *Science* 298(5599):1694–5.

Pennisi E. 2003. Reaching their goals early, sequencing labs celebrate. *Science* 300(5618):409.

Pressman L. 2002. AUTM Licensing Survey: FY 2000. See <www.autm.net>.

Rettig RA. 1977. Cancer Crusade: The Story of the National Cancer Act of 1971. Princeton, NJ: Princeton University Press.

Roberts L. 2002. Genome research. A tussle over the rules for DNA data sharing. *Science* 298(5597):1312–3.

Rossouw JE, Finnegan LP, Harlan WR, Pinn VW, Clifford C, McGowan JA. 1995. The evolution of the Women's Health Initiative: perspectives from the NIH. *J Am Med Womens Assoc* 50(2):50–5.

Rossouw JE, Anderson GL, Prentice RL, LaCroix AZ, Kooperberg C, Stefanick ML, Jackson RD, Beresford SA, Howard BV, Johnson KC, Kotchen JM, Ockene J. 2002. Risks and benefits of estrogen plus progestin in healthy postmenopausal women: principal results from the Women's Health Initiative randomized controlled trial. *JAMA* 288(3):321–33.

Rowen L, Mahairas G, Hood L. 1997. Sequencing the human genome. *Science* 278(5338): 605–7.

Sachidanandam R, Weissman D, Schmidt SC, Kakol JM, Stein LD, Marth G, Sherry S, Mullikin JC, Mortimore BJ, Willey DL, Hunt SE, Cole CG, Coggill PC, Rice CM, Ning Z, Rogers J, Bentley DR, Kwok PY, Mardis ER, Yeh RT, Schultz B, Cook L, Davenport R, Dante M, Fulton L, Hillier L, Waterston RH, McPherson JD, Gilman B, Schaffner S, Van Etten WJ, Reich D, Higgins J, Daly MJ, Blumenstiel B, Baldwin J, Stange-Thomann

N, Zody MC, Linton L, Lander ES, Atshuler D. 2001. A map of human genome sequence variation containing 1.42 million single nucleotide polymorphisms. *Nature* 409(6822):928–33.

Science and Government Alert. Zerhouni presents road map for NIH's future to his advisors. December 13, 2002. Washington, DC.

ScienceScope. 2000. Relishing victory. *Science* 288(5474):2299.

ScienceScope. 2002. *Science* 295(5562):1991.

Service RF. 2000. Proteomics. Can Celera do it again? *Science* 287(5461):2136–8.

Service RF. 2001a. Proteomics. A proteomics upstart tries to outrun the competition. *Science* 294(5549):2079–80.

Service RF. 2001b. Proteomics. Gene and protein patents get ready to go head to head. *Science* 294(5549):2082–3.

Service RF. 2001c. Proteomics. High-speed biologists search for gold in proteins. *Science* 294(5549):2074–7.

Service RF. 2002. Structural genomics. Tapping DNA for structures produces a trickle. *Science* 298(5595):948–50.

Shine KI. 1998. Encouraging clinical research by physician scientists. *JAMA* 280:1442–4.

Smaglik P. 2000. Genomics initiative to decipher 10,000 protein structures. *Nature* 407(6804): 549.

Smaglik P. 2001. Building Protein Pipelines. *Nature (Naturejobs)*.413(6851):4–6.

Softcheck J. 2002. Federal R&D at $111.8 billion in President's FY 03 budget proposal, Marburger says. Washington, DC: Washington Fax.

Spieler R. 2002. NIH works to protect research data from incursion while pressing researchers to share among themselves. Washington, DC: Washington Fax.

Stephan PE, Black G. 2001. Bioinformatics: Emerging opportunities and emerging gaps, In: Capitalizing on New Needs and New Opportunities: Government—Industry Partnerships in Biotechnology and Information Technologies. Washington, DC: National Academy Press.

Stevens RC, Yokoyama S, Wilson IA. 2001. Global efforts in structural genomics. *Science* 294(5540):89–92.

Stockwell BR. 2000. Chemical genetics: ligand-based discovery of gene function. *Nat Rev Genet* 1(2):116–25.

Sulston J, Ferry G. 2002. The Common Thread: A Story of Science, Politics, Ethics, and the Human Genome. 1st ed. Washington, DC: Joseph Henry Press.

Task Force on the Future of Clinician Scientists at UCSF. 2000. The Future of Clinician Scientists: Initial Report and Recommendations. San Francisco, CA: UCSF.

Thomas P, Gilbert D. 2002. Opinion. Beyond Serendipity. *The Scientist* 16(23):12.

Thorner B. 1997. Trading patent rights for research tools: What's at stake? *Nat Biotechnol* 15(10):1024–27.

UCOP (University of California Office of the President). 1997. Tenure review.

U.S. Congress General Accounting Office. 1999. August. Technology Transfer: Reporting Requirements for Federally Sponsored Inventions Need Revision: Washington, DC: General Accounting Office.

U.S. Department of Health, Education, and Welfare. 1966. Report of the Secretary's Advisory Committee on the Management of National Institutes of Health Research Contracts and Grants. (Ruina Report). Washington, DC: Government Printing Office.

U.S. Department of Health, Education, and Welfare. 1973. National Cancer Program. Report of the National Cancer Advisory Board. Washington, DC: Government Printing Office. Notes: DHEW Publication No. (NIH) 74–471.

U.S. Department of Health and Human Services, Office of the Inspector General. 1994. NIH Oversight of Extramural Research Inventions. Washington, DC: Department of Health and Human Services.

U.S. Patent and Trademark Office. 2000. Performance and Accountability Report, Fiscal Year 2000. Washington, DC: USPTO.

U.S. President's NIH Study Committee. 1965. Biomedical Science and Its Administration: A Study of the National Institutes of Health. Report to the President. (Wooldridge Committee Report). Washington, DC: Government Printing Office.

Varmus H. 1998. New Directions in Biology and Medicine. Philadelphia, PA.

Varmus H. 1999. Evaluating the burden of disease and spending the research dollars of the National Institutes of Health. *N Engl J Med* 340:1914–5.

Varmus H. 2001. Public health. Proliferation of National Institutes of Health. *Science* 291(5510): 1903–5.

Venter JC, Adams MD, Myers EW, Li PW, Mural RJ, Sutton GG, Smith HO, Yandell M, Evans CA, Holt RA, Gocayne JD, Amanatides P, Ballew RM, Huson DH, Wortman JR, Zhang Q, Kodira CD, Zheng XH, Chen L, Skupski M, Subramanian G, Thomas PD, Zhang J, Gabor Miklos GL, Nelson C, Broder S, Clark AG, Nadeau J, McKusick VA, Zinder N, Levine AJ, Roberts RJ, Simon M, Slayman C, Hunkapiller M, Bolanos R, Delcher A, Dew I, Fasulo D, Flanigan M, Florea L, Halpern A, Hannenhalli S, Kravitz S, Levy S, Mobarry C, Reinert K, Remington K, Abu-Threideh J, Beasley E, Biddick K, Bonazzi V, Brandon R, Cargill M, Chandramouliswaran I, Charlab R, Chaturvedi K, Deng Z, Di Francesco V, Dunn P, Eilbeck K, Evangelista C, Gabrielian AE, Gan W, Ge W, Gong F, Gu Z, Guan P, Heiman TJ, Higgins ME, Ji RR, Ke Z, Ketchum KA, Lai Z, Lei Y, Li Z, Li J, Liang Y, Lin X, Lu F, Merkulov GV, Milshina N, Moore HM, Naik AK, Narayan VA, Neelam B, Nusskern D, Rusch DB, Salzberg S, Shao W, Shue B, Sun J, Wang Z, Wang A, Wang X, Wang J, Wei M, Wides R, Xiao C, Yan C, Yao A, Ye J, Zhan M, Zhang W, Zhang H, Zhao Q, Zheng L, Zhong F, Zhong W, Zhu S, Zhao S, Gilbert D, Baumhueter S, Spier G, Carter C, Cravchik A, Woodage T, Ali F, An H, Awe A, Baldwin D, Baden H, Barnstead M, Barrow I, Beeson K, Busam D, Carver A, Center A, Cheng ML, Curry L, Danaher S, Davenport L, Desilets R, Dietz S, Dodson K, Doup L, Ferriera S, Garg N, Gluecksmann A, Hart B, Haynes J, Haynes C, Heiner C, Hladun S, Hostin D, Houck J, Howland T, Ibegwam C, Johnson J, Kalush F, Kline L, Koduru S, Love A, Mann F, May D, McCawley S, McIntosh T, McMullen I, Moy M, Moy L, Murphy B, Nelson K, Pfannkoch C, Pratts E, Puri V, Qureshi H, Reardon M, Rodriguez R, Rogers YH, Romblad D, Ruhfel B, Scott R, Sitter C, Smallwood M, Stewart E, Strong R, Suh E, Thomas R, Tint NN, Tse S, Vech C, Wang G, Wetter J, Williams S, Williams M, Windsor S, Winn-Deen E, Wolfe K, Zaveri J, Zaveri K, Abril JF, Guigo R, Campbell MJ, Sjolander KV, Karlak B, Kejariwal A, Mi H, Lazareva B, Hatton T, Narechania A, Diemer K, Muruganujan A, Guo N, Sato S, Bafna V, Istrail S, Lippert R, Schwartz R, Walenz B, Yooseph S, Allen D, Basu A, Baxendale J, Blick L, Caminha M, Carnes-Stine J, Caulk P, Chiang YH, Coyne M, Dahlke C, Mays A, Dombroski M, Donnelly M, Ely D, Esparham S, Fosler C, Gire H, Glanowski S, Glasser K, Glodek A, Gorokhov M, Graham K, Gropman B, Harris M, Heil J, Henderson S, Hoover J, Jennings D, Jordan C, Jordan J, Kasha J, Kagan L, Kraft C, Levitsky A, Lewis M, Liu X, Lopez J, Ma D, Majoros W, McDaniel J, Murphy S, Newman M, Nguyen T, Nguyen N, Nodell M, Pan S, Peck J, Peterson M, Rowe W, Sanders R, Scott J, Simpson M, Smith T, Sprague A, Stockwell T, Turner R, Venter E, Wang M, Wen M, Wu D, Wu M, Xia A, Zandieh A, Zhu X. 2001. The sequence of the human genome. *Science* 291(5507):1304–51.

Venter JC, Adams MD, Sutton GG, Kerlavage AR, Smith HO, Hunkapiller M. 1998. Shotgun sequencing of the human genome. *Science* 280(5369):1540–2.

Vogel G. 1999. A day in the life of a topflight lab. *Science* 285(5433):1531–2.

Wade N. 2001. Life Script: How the Human Genome Discoveries Will Transform Medicine and Enhance Your Health. New York: Simon & Schuster.

Warner S. 2002. Once promising proteomics market sags. *The Scientist* 16(8):18.

Washington Fax. 2001. DOE lab signs joint venture with Celera and Compaq to create biology supercomputers. Washington, DC: Washington Fax.

Waterston RH, Lander ES, Sulston JE. 2002a. On the sequencing of the human genome. *Proc Natl Acad Sci USA* 99:3712–6.

Waterston RH, Lindblad-Toh K, Birney E, Rogers J, Abril JF, Agarwal P, Agarwala R, Ainscough R, Alexandersson M, An P, Antonarakis SE, Attwood J, Baertsch R, Bailey J, Barlow K, Beck S, Berry E, Birren B, Bloom T, Bork P, Botcherby M, Bray N, Brent MR, Brown DG, Brown SD, Bult C, Burton J, Butler J, Campbell RD, Carninci P, Cawley S, Chiaromonte F, Chinwalla AT, Church DM, Clamp M, Clee C, Collins FS, Cook LL, Copley RR, Coulson A, Couronne O, Cuff J, Curwen V, Cutts T, Daly M, David R, Davies J, Delehaunty KD, Deri J, Dermitzakis ET, Dewey C, Dickens NJ, Diekhans M, Dodge S, Dubchak I, Dunn DM, Eddy SR, Elnitski L, Emes RD, Eswara P, Eyras E, Felsenfeld A, Fewell GA, Flicek P, Foley K, Frankel WN, Fulton LA, Fulton RS, Furey TS, Gage D, Gibbs RA, Glusman G, Gnerre S, Goldman N, Goodstadt L, Grafham D, Graves TA, Green ED, Gregory S, Guigo R, Guyer M, Hardison RC, Haussler D, Hayashizaki Y, Hillier LW, Hinrichs A, Hlavina W, Holzer T, Hsu F, Hua A, Hubbard T, Hunt A, Jackson I, Jaffe DB, Johnson LS, Jones M, Jones TA, Joy A, Kamal M, Karlsson EK, Karolchik D, Kasprzyk A, Kawai J, Keibler E, Kells C, Kent WJ, Kirby A, Kolbe DL, Korf I, Kucherlapati RS, Kulbokas EJ, Kulp D, Landers T, Leger JP, Leonard S, Letunic I, Levine R, Li J, Li M, Lloyd C, Lucas S, Ma B, Maglott DR, Mardis ER, Matthews L, Mauceli E, Mayer JH, McCarthy M, McCombie WR, McLaren S, McLay K, McPherson JD, Meldrim J, Meredith B, Mesirov JP, Miller W, Miner TL, Mongin E, Montgomery KT, Morgan M, Mott R, Mullikin JC, Muzny DM, Nash WE, Nelson JO, Nhan MN, Nicol R, Ning Z, Nusbaum C, O'Connor MJ, Okazaki Y, Oliver K, Overton-Larty E, Pachter L, Parra G, Pepin KH, Peterson J, Pevzner P, Plumb R, Pohl CS, Poliakov A, Ponce TC, Ponting CP, Potter S, Quail M, Reymond A, Roe BA, Roskin KM, Rubin EM, Rust AG, Santos R, Sapojnikov V, Schultz B, Schultz J, Schwartz MS, Schwartz S, Scott C, Seaman S, Searle S, Sharpe T, Sheridan A, Shownkeen R, Sims S, Singer JB, Slater G, Smit A, Smith DR, Spencer B, Stabenau A, Stange-Thomann N, Sugnet C, Suyama M, Tesler G, Thompson J, Torrents D, Trevaskis E, Tromp J, Ucla C, Ureta-Vidal A, Vinson JP, Von Niederhausern AC, Wade CM, Wall M, Weber RJ, Weiss RB, Wendl MC, West AP, Wetterstrand K, Wheeler R, Whelan S, Wierzbowski J, Willey D, Williams S, Wilson RK, Winter E, Worley KC, Wyman D, Yang S, Yang SP, Zdobnov EM, Zody MC, Lander ES. 2002b. Initial sequencing and comparative analysis of the mouse genome. *Nature* 420(6915):520–62.

Wessely S, Wood F. 1999. Peer Review of Grant Applications: A Systematic Review. Peer Review in Health Sciences. Annapolis Junction, MD: BMJ Publishing Group.

Yoshida M, Miyoshi I, Hinuma Y. 1982. Isolation and characterization of retrovirus from cell lines of human adult T-cell leukemia and its implication in the disease. *Proc Natl Acad Sci USA* 79:2031–5.

Zemlo TR, Garrison HH, Partridge NC, Ley TJ. 2000. The Physician Scientist: Career Issues and Challenges at the Year 2000. Bethesda, MD: FASEB Life Sciences Forum. Pp. 14:221.

Appendix

A History of Government Funding of Basic Science Research and the Development of Big-Science Projects in the Context of High-Energy Particle Physics

MaryJoy Ballantyne
Research Associate
National Cancer Policy Board
Institute of Medicine
The National Academies

Contents

Since World War II, the organizational framework for scientific research is increasingly the multi-institutional collaboration. However, this form of research has received slight attention from scholars. Without a dedicated effort to understand such collaborations, policy makers and administrators will continue to have only hearsay and their own memories to guide their management....
(AIP, 1992)

This paper is a supplement to a study conducted by the National Cancer Policy Board on big science in cancer research. As the study committee ventured out in search of the available literature to address the issues in our tentative outline, including how large-scale projects should best be prioritized, funded, organized, managed, and staffed, we received an abundance of verbal and editorial affirmations regarding these issues and the direction we were taking, but no analytical scholarship. To date, no studies have been conducted in the biological sciences to address the questions we are asking. Instead, we were repeatedly referred to the field of high-energy particle physics—the field that inspired Alvin Weinberg to coin the phrase "big science" in 1961 (Weinberg, 1961). The origins of the field of high-energy particle physics, as well as the evolution of federal investment in science research, can be traced back to before World War II. During our study of this field, we found a wealth of interesting and helpful historical summaries, papers, surveys, and thoughtful analyses that address directly or indirectly several of the issues the Board has associated with big science in cancer research.

This paper is divided into two major sections. The first is a brief account of the organization of a group of key federal regulatory and funding agencies that have influenced the formation of current federal science and technology policy. This account is presented in the form of a selected chronological history of the government's earliest support for basic and applied science research, both intramural and extramural, leading up to university-based publicly funded research. Though the section is outlined as a chronology according to the agencies' founding date, there is noticeable but unavoidable overlap in several of the subsections. The second section examines several of the issues unique to the development, pursuit, implementation, and practice of big-science projects in the field of high-energy particle physics, as indicated by scientists and policy makers associated with that field.

PART I: HISTORY OF GOVERNMENT FUNDING OF UNIVERSITY-BASED BASIC SCIENCE RESEARCH, EDUCATION, AND TRAINING

It has been basic United States policy that government should foster the opening of new frontiers. It opened the seas to clipper ships and furnished land for pioneers. Although these frontiers have more or less disappeared, the frontier of science remains. It is in keeping with the American tradition—one which has made the United States great—that new frontiers shall be made accessible for development by all American citizens. (Bush, 1945b)

Traditionally, the U.S. government has used its resources to pursue matters of national importance. As the country's foundations were being laid, the nation relied very little on matters of science. Though U.S. scientific pursuits had a slow start, strong foundations were formed early in the nineteenth century through federally sponsored research programs in agriculture, national security, and commerce that facilitated significant momentum in government sponsorship of public-based scientific endeavors in the early part of the twentieth century. It should be noted that before the surge of federal funds into public research programs, private philanthropic foundations, such as Carnegie, Rockefeller, and Smithsonian, provided much of the earliest support for university-based basic research. This was definitely true for the field of high-energy particle physics, which received most of its initial support from such foundations as Rockefeller and Carnegie (Heilbron et al., 1981).

Pre-World War II

In the United States, the period of time closely preceding, including, and following World War II had a significant impact on the government's investment in university-based scientific research. During the decade surrounding the war, from 1940 to 1950, various key people and events facilitated the creation and expansion of several science-oriented federal agencies whose main objective was sponsoring public research, thus enabling the expansion of federal policy regarding science research. The foundation for these developments had been laid during the previous century through the government's involvement in a variety of science research programs in the areas of exploration, agriculture, security, and settlement, though most of these initial programs were intramural in nature. These pursuits led to the organization of a few federal agencies that conducted or sponsored science research, including the U.S. Coast Survey, the Department of Agriculture, and the U.S. Geological Survey. Although the government hired civil scientists to assist and conduct research on these federal projects prior to World War II, it allocated little funding directly to universities in support of scientific education, training, and basic research. During and directly after World War II, federal science policy was created and refined into the federal funding of university-based scientific research, which continued to evolve to form the substantial endowment that has become the accepted and expected norm today.

1787: The Constitutional Convention

The idea that the federal government should become the patron of science was easily within the grasp of the framers of the Constitution, which was written by educated men who held all branches of philosophy in high regard, and who knew that European governments often supported science. As they went about their political task of writing the Constitution, they gave consideration and debate to the constitutional position of science with regard to the federal government they were establishing. Debate ensued during the Constitutional Convention of the late 1780s, as proposals outlining government's relationship with science were presented. Proposals for a national university devoted to advanced scientific training, societies chartered by the government, technical schools, and prized and direct subsidies for creative effort could all have become realities. Because of a fear of powerful central organizations, the consensus was to restrict the powers of the central government. The Constitution, ratified in April 1789, contained very little language directly related to science. However, it did include the concepts of "internal improvements," "general welfare," and "necessary and proper," as well as a clause for patents that gave Congress power to "promote the Progress of Science and useful Arts, by securing for limited Times to Authors and Inventors the exclusive Right to their respective Writings and Discoveries" (Dupree, 1986). It was through these fragments of language that the federal government would eventually support and sustain science.

After ratification, interpretation of the Constitution began, and public works of all sorts were inferred from the concept of "internal improvements." During this time, most highly educated Americans had obtained a university education in Europe and were still dependent on Europe for equipment and ideas. Despite the debates, all sides agreed that universities and learned societies were in fact internal improvements, and that they were necessary and proper and sustained the general welfare. The idea of a national university was emphatically pursued by many, but never came to fruition. One of the most avid supporters of this idea was Thomas Jefferson, who was secretary of state; he would soon become responsible for administering U.S. patents, which would be the earliest connection between science and the federal government.

Although the framers explicitly avoided the word "patent," the qualifying phrases in the language of the Constitution suggest the English practice of protecting new inventions for a limited time (Dupree, 1986). As a result of confusion surrounding this language, Congress passed the first patent act in 1790 at the request of President Washington. The secretaries of state and of war and the attorney general constituted a board to pass on inventions. The board had full authority to refuse patents because of a lack of novelty, utility, or importance, which placed the heavy responsibility of making technical decisions on three of the four leading men in Washington (Dupree, 1986).

Jefferson, administrator of the patent law of 1790, disliked monopolies of all kinds, including patents of limited duration, but came to see the latter's usefulness as a grant from society to encourage inventors by giving them some chance of receiving a financial return for their work (Dupree, 1986). Jefferson upheld a strict interpretation of the law, according to which patents had to be real novelties, not familiar devices or principles common to the public. Thus a principle abstracted from a machine was not patentable, only the device itself. These assumptions had two very important influences on Jefferson's administration of the patent law. First, science itself was rigidly excluded from patents. Second, and paradoxically, all the techniques of science were to be applied by the government to a patent application in an active effort to protect the public from unwarranted exclusiveness. Jefferson's personal contributions to and understanding and veneration of science allowed him to take these initial steps connecting the federal government with science, while at the same time protecting science from the federal government.

Jefferson's influence on linking science and the federal government would lead to the creation of the first federal science project—the Coast Survey. Through all the twists and turns of U.S. political history, and through the immense changes wrought by over two centuries of rapidly expanding scientific knowledge, the policies and activities of the government in science form a single strand that connects the Constitutional Convention to current science policy (Dupree, 1986).

1807: Survey of the Coast

The earliest American pursuits in government-funded science research began in the military. Congress did not authorize civilian scientific activities in the federal government until 1807, when, with the support of President Thomas Jefferson, it established the Coast Survey for the practical purpose of providing better charts of coastal waters and navigational aids for commercial interests. The Coast Survey could not get under way until after the end of the War of 1812, when it was transferred several times between the Department of the Treasury (1816–1818, 1832–1834, 1836–1903) and the Navy (1818–1832, 1834–1836). It became the U.S. Coast and Geodetic Survey and was transferred in 1913 to the Department of Commerce, where it was later consolidated with the National Weather Service, and where it currently resides as part of the National Oceanic and Atmospheric Administration (NOAA) (Rabbitt, 2000; U.S. National Oceanic and Atmospheric Administration, 2001).

As is true of most successful ventures, the Coast Survey's significant contributions to the advancement and development of American science can be attributed largely to an influential leader. In 1843, Alexander Dallas Bache, a great-grandson of Benjamin Franklin, took the helm of the project. He had the ability to work within the American political scene for the benefit of both the Coast Survey and American science. The project prospered during his tenure as superintendent, becoming the first great science organization of the U.S. government. Bache embarked on a policy of publishing the results of the Coast Survey and the related work of other professional scientists in the *Annual Report of the Superintendent of the Coast Survey*, elevating American science in the eyes of the world scientific community (*Coast and Geodetic Survey Annual Reports, 1844–1910*). His accomplishments in promoting science included his service in the organization of the American Association for the Advancement of Science (AAAS) and as a founder of the National Academy of Sciences (NAS).

The early years of the Coast Survey reflect the growth of nineteenth-century American physical science, including rapid advances in knowledge and technology in several fields of earth sciences, including geodesy, geophysics, hydrography, topography, and oceanography. Early work on the project also generated a number of noteworthy published papers in the fields of astronomy, geology, and meteorology. Almost as a precedent for today's technology momentum, the gain in basic knowledge made through the work of the Survey spurred technological developments that made it possible to facilitate geographic exploration; implement harbor improvements; advance printing, engraving, and photographic technology; and strengthen national defense. The benefits and success of this scientific endeavor made the initial influence of a federally sponsored science program on national science policy and politics a positive one, enabling the expansion of federal support within the nation's science-oriented programs. The forerunner of today's National Institute of Standards and Technology resided within the Coast and Geodetic Survey (*Coast and Geodetic Survey Annual Reports, 1844–1910*).

Work on the Coast Survey spanned the continental United States, tying together travel between the east and west coasts. Through precise nautical charting surveys, American commerce began to flourish as commercial ships were led more safely into ports all along the Atlantic, Gulf, and Pacific shores. Under Superintendent Bache, contributors to the Survey in both the field and the office were held to the highest standard of accuracy in obtaining and recording scientific measurements. The office force consisted of a wide range of professionals, including mathematicians, physicists, geodesists, astronomers, instrument makers, draftsmen, engravers, and pressmen.

Scientific contributions attributed to the Coast Survey include highly accurate astronomic measurements, new and more accurate observational instrumentation for sea and land surveying, new techniques for mathematical analysis of the data obtained in the field, and further-refined techniques for error analysis and mitigation. It was the Coast Survey that led American science away from the older descriptive scientific methods to the current techniques of statistical analysis and the use of mathematical modeling to predict future states of natural phenomena (*Coast and Geodetic Survey Annual Reports, 1844–1910*). In addition, during its early tenure within the Navy, the Coast Survey conducted activities that led to the establishment of the Depot of Charts and Instruments in 1844, which served as a central office where both naval and commercial seamen could deposit and retrieve new navigational information and technology. In the mid-1800s, this office was divided into the Naval Observatory and the Naval Hydrographic Office, whose respective responsibilities included gathering astronomical data for navigation and charting the ocean floor (National Archives and Records Administration Records of the Coast and Geodetic Survey, 1807–1965).

1862: The Department of Agriculture and The Land Grant College Acts

Agriculture has always been a national priority, and was an occupation in one form or another for many U.S. citizens during the 1800s. The usefulness of science for economic purposes in the field of agriculture was documented in May 1862, when Congress established the Department of Agriculture "to acquire and diffuse... useful information on subjects connected with agriculture," and authorized "practical and scientific experiments" to obtain this information (Rabbitt, 2000). To this end, the Land Grant College Acts, also known as the Morrill Acts of 1862 and 1890, were signed into law by President Abraham Lincoln. The acts initiated one of the first programs of federal support for university-based basic research. The first act requested that the federal government provide each state with a grant of land that could be sold to finance a college—hence the term "land-grant." The second act provided direct appropriations to land-grant colleges that could show that race and color were not admission criteria. These acts allowed members of the working classes to obtain a liberal, practical education in such areas as agriculture, military tactics, and mechanical arts, as well as classical studies.

Several other pieces of legislation further defined land-grant colleges. The Hatch Act of 1887 authorized $15,000 for direct payment of federal grant funds to each state for the establishment of an agricultural experiment station in connection with the state's land-grant institution (Rosenberg, 1997; IFAS, 2000). The funds were provided to enable the colleges to conduct agricultural research and pursue scientific knowledge that could be shared with students and farmers. Unfortunately, many university administrators saw the Hatch Act as a windfall for undernourished academic funds, and misused its appropriations to pay salaries and other university expenses. The Department of Agriculture set up the Office of Experiment Stations (OES) to regulate and review the activities of the stations, but it took several years for this new office to develop a sound and well-articulated policy ensuring that the Hatch appropriations would be used as a research fund. The original wording of the Hatch Act was ultimately unsatisfactory as an administrative tool to control station research policies and as a source of funds to support basic research.

The Adams Act of 1906 took the Hatch Act a bit further, gradually increasing each state's appropriation to $30,000, this sum to be used exclusively for "original investigation(s)" in scientific research (Rosenberg, 1997). To ensure that stations and universities would comply with the Adams Act, OES established a new administrative tool now known as the grant system; all plans for conducting research with the Adams appropriations had to be submitted as a proposal for approval before the work itself could be undertaken. The development of the grants system, along with the research conducted by the stations, played a substantial role in the development of a number of biological sciences in the United States, including bacteriology, biochemistry, and genetics (Goldberg, 1995). The Smith-Lever Act of 1914 extended the concept of service to the community by creating the federal Cooperative Extension Service.

These measures contributed to the creation and success of many of the country's well-known universities, including Purdue University, Massachusetts Institute of Technology (MIT), Rutgers University, Cornell University, the University of Wisconsin, Texas A&M University, and Iowa State University. The later success of the land-grant colleges was due, in part, to experimental farms, which grew out of the experiment stations. The achievements of these farms include improvements in fertilizers, seed corn, pesticides, fruits, livestock breeding, and disease control. Today there are 105 land-grant colleges and universities, including those in U.S. territories such as Guam and the Virgin Islands and 29 Native American institutions.

1870: United States Weather Service

At about the same time as the development of the land-grant colleges, civilian and military weather observation networks began to grow and expand across the United States. The telegraph was largely responsible for the advancement of operational meteorology during the nineteenth century. With the advent of the telegraph, weather observations from distant points could be rapidly collected, plotted, and analyzed at one location. These weather services were hosted by several independent networks and lacked a central storage and dissemination facility.

With the support of several meteorological physicists, and in keeping with the nation's interest in agriculture, national security, and commerce, Congress established a national weather warning service in 1870, which was purposely organized within the Army Signal Corps under the Secretary of War to ensure the greatest promptness, regularity, and accuracy. President Grant authorized "the secretary of War to take observations at military stations and to warn of storms on the Great Lakes and on the Atlantic and Gulf Coasts" (Grice, 2001). Two years later, this forecast service was extended throughout the United States. The Signal Service's field stations grew in number from 24 in 1870 to 284 in 1878. Each station telegraphed an observation to Washington, D.C., at three designated times during the day. Washington compiled forecasts from the telegraph reports, which were then distributed throughout the country (Grice, 2001).

During the first 20 years of the weather service, research studies were conducted at the central office in Washington, D.C. The initial meteorology research program, largely intramural, was conducted by a team of about eight scientists, and included studies on the distribution of moisture in the air, a treatise on the laws of meteorology, a report on tornadoes, and instructional material for Signal Service trainees. In 1890, after a raucous embezzlement scandal, the Signal Service was transferred out of the army to the Department of Agriculture, where it became the civilian Weather Bureau, began to publish daily weather maps, and established a hurricane warning service. In 1940 the service was again transferred, this time to the Department of Commerce, where it issued the first official daily forecasts. The service was eventually combined with the U.S. Coast and Geodetic Survey and renamed the National Weather Service. The National Weather Service, which currently resides under the jurisdiction of NOAA, provides the bulk of all meteorological information used in forecasting weather conditions both inside and outside of the United States.

As the benefits of weather prediction became obvious in the areas of agriculture, commerce, and defense, the need for more extensive and more accurate forecasting became a national priority. The federal investment in the young weather service and in skilled scientists produced important new knowledge and technology. In so doing, it represented another positive contribution that strengthened the federal policy of supporting scientific research programs. The beneficial effect of the government's role in the acquisition, application, and dissemination of scientific knowledge was becoming more apparent and necessary. Also increasingly apparent was the interdependence between the knowledge base gained in basic science research and the growth and availability of technology.

1879: U.S. Geological Survey

The earliest geological surveys were conducted mainly in support of agriculture, which was the basic occupation in the United States throughout most of the nineteenth century. These first surveys were generally sponsored by independent state or local governments. With the conclusion of the Civil War, the federal government, in need of an accurate assessment of its western territories, incorporated the investigation, mapping, and understanding of these territories into its domestic policy (PBS, 1999). The U.S. Government wanted to know whether the land could be farmed, what its natural resources were, and how easily it could be settled. From 1867 to 1879, Congress began to sponsor what became known as the four Great Surveys. These surveys predated the formation of the U.S. Geological Survey. Each was a large undertaking in terms of both the amount of territory they examined and the wealth of information they contributed to the knowledge of the American West (PBS, 1999).

One of the first surveys was directed by Dr. Ferdinand Vandeveer Hayden. Hayden's expedition initially came under the supervision of the General Land Office and, despite its modest start, became the largest of the Great Surveys. With an initial appropriation of $5,000, Hayden's original commission was to explore the lands of Nebraska, investigating areas of the state suitable for human exploitation. Within 2 years, his annual appropriation had doubled, his investigation had been formally titled The United States Geological Survey of the Territories, and his work had been placed under the authority of the Secretary of the Interior. Hayden's most ambitious expeditions were the well-equipped investigations of the Yellowstone and Teton Mountain area of Wyoming. The photographs and drawings he brought back to Washington from those trips assisted legislators in creating Yellowstone National Park. Hayden moved his investigations to Colorado, a transition that would put him in direct confrontation with another surveying team. Ultimately, Hayden's survey was important in a number of ways. In addition to mapping the West, it provided a wealth of knowledge about the region's natural history, and the artists, photographers, and newspaper reporters who accompanied his teams helped demystify the western territories for Americans (Rabbitt, 2000).

The year Hayden's operation was established, 25-year-old Clarence King, an affluent aristocrat from New England, arrived in Washington with a handful of recommendations from scientists and the desire to direct his own survey in the western territories. His plan was to survey a 100-mile-wide belt along the 40th parallel that would roughly follow the route of the transcontinental railway. Upon granting King his commission—an expedition entitled the Geological Survey of the Fortieth Parallel—the secretary of war dispensed some advice: "The sooner you get out of Washington, the better. You are too young a man to be seen about town with this appointment in your pocket. There are four major-generals who want your place" (Rabbitt, 2000).

King was a cautious and meticulous scholar. Unlike Hayden, who believed that any discoveries should immediately be made known to the public, King decided that his reports would represent the careful distillation of years of research: "It is my intention to give this work a finish which will place it on an equal footing with the best European productions" (Rabbitt, 2000). To do this, King hired the best geologists and staffed the survey with first-rate scientists, including topographers, geologists, botanists, and an ornithologist. The survey's research program extended beyond geology to include studies in paleontology, botany, and ornithology. The seven-volume report and accompanying atlas of the 40th parallel that resulted from the investigation did much to improve the reputation of American science in Europe. King's own contribution, *Systematic Geology,* was for decades a classic historical geological text. When it was published in 1878, it was the most comprehensive thesis to date on the subject (Rabbitt, 2000).

In 1867, the same year that Hayden and King approached Congress for financial support for their surveys, John Wesley Powell, a one-armed Civil War veteran, was also seeking sponsorship of an expedition. He secured nothing more than the promise of some wagons, livestock, camp equipment, and surveying gadgets. After his famous and successful first expedition down the Colorado River in 1869, Powell was granted a congressional appropriation to "complete the survey of the Colorado of the West and its tributaries" (Rabbitt, 2000). Powell concentrated his investigations on a narrow rectangular area bordered by the Green River and the Uinta Mountains in the north, the Grand Canyon in the south, and Colorado in the west. Of all the Great Surveys, Powell's was initially staffed by men with the least knowledge and expertise. The initial work of the survey, including the river trip and an exploration of the Great Plateau, was concluded by 1873. For the next 6 years, a handful of professional men remained in the field continuing the survey work, while Powell spent most of these years in Washington, D.C. His survey focused on geology, and although it did not produce the volumes of published material that emerged from the other surveys, it made important contributions in its explanations of the formation of the Grand Canyon's geological features, which helped open up new areas of geological investigation.

In 1871, the Army Corps of Engineers inaugurated its own survey, initiated in part because of a belief within the army that civilians were usurping its traditional, pre–Civil War, peacetime activity of mapmaking. The army claimed that no one else was making maps suitable for military purposes. Lieutenant George Montague Wheeler was put in charge of the fourth Great Survey—the Geographical Surveys West of the 100th Meridian—to obtain "correct topographical knowledge of the region traversed . . . and to prepare accurate maps of that section" (Rabbitt, 2000). Additionally, he was required to determine "everything relating to the physical features of the country, the numbers, habits, and disposition of the Indians who may live in this section . . . and the facilities offered for making rail or common roads, to meet the wants of those who at some future period may occupy or traverse this portion of our territory" (Rabbitt, 2000).

By the early 1870s, there were four different investigations of overlapping territory; conflict was inevitable. In 1872, Powell began campaigning to consolidate the work of the surveys. But Congress took no notice of the rivalries and needless duplication until Hayden's and Wheeler's men clashed in the Colorado territory in July 1873. Shortly thereafter, the House of Representatives held hearings into whether the survey work should be collapsed into one larger survey. The proceedings were notable for a succession of bitter and angry complaints. Faced with conflicting opinions from the various expedition leaders, Congress decided that all the surveys should continue.

In 1878, Powell again lobbied for the consolidation of the three remaining surveys. In June of that year, NAS was asked to consider the issue. The resulting report suggested consolidating the investigations under the supervision of the Department of the Interior. A new agency, the U.S. Geological Survey, was established in 1879 to carry out the work. King was hired as its first director. Within a year he had stepped down and been replaced by Powell, who would head the organization for the next 23 years. Over the next century, the U.S. Geological Survey became firmly incorporated into the federal government. Today its many activities include predicting earthquakes, evaluating water quality, and producing tens of thousands of maps (PBS, 1999; Rabbitt, 2000).

1887: The National Institutes of Health (NIH)

NIH began in an attic room in the Marine Hospital in Stapleton on Staten Island, New York. Dr. Joseph Kinyoun (1860–1919), a 27-year-old bacteriologist and graduate of Bellevue Hospital Medical College in New

York City, who had been instrumental in introducing the production of diphtheria and tetanus antitoxin serums in the United States, set up his one-person Laboratory of Hygiene as the federal government's first research institution. The laboratory's purpose was to identify and seek cures for infectious diseases, as well as to tackle other public health problems. In 1891, the laboratory needed more space and was moved to Washington, D.C., and renamed the Hygienic Laboratory. Further change came to the Hygienic Laboratory in 1930. Its continued progress, illustrated by 45 years of successful research that resulted in the comprehensive identification and analysis of Rocky Mountain spotted fever, convinced Senator Joseph E. Randsell of Louisiana that fundamental research could lead to cures for disease (NIH, 2001). The Randsell Act was passed by Congress to reorganize and expand the Hygienic Laboratory and change its name to the National Institute of Health. In 1938, a continually growing National Institute of Health began its move from Washington, D.C., to suburban Bethesda, Maryland (Rettig, 1977).

World War II marked a change in the basic research conducted by the National Institute of Health. The scope of its investigations was broadened to include fundamental medical research on major chronic diseases, such as cancer, cardiovascular disease, arthritis, and mental illness. It was also at this time that the extramural research program began with the transfer of certain wartime medical research contracts from the Office of Scientific Research and Development (OSRD; see below). In 1948 four institutes were created to support work on cardiac disease, dental disorders, infectious diseases, and experimental biology and medicine, and the National Institute of Health (singular) officially became the National Institutes of Health (plural). In that same year, construction began on the Clinical Center, a hospital with over 500 beds, which was designed to facilitate the development of therapies (NIH, 2001; Rettig, 1977).

1916: The Naval Research Laboratory (NRL)

Throughout the nineteenth century and in the early twentieth century, the U.S. military depended heavily on the navy. To ensure the nation's security, it was necessary for the navy to remain current with developing technologies. At the outset of the World War I, Thomas Edison suggested that "the Government should maintain a great research laboratory.... In this could be developed ... all the technique of military and naval progression without vast expense" (NRL, 2001). Among elite scientists of the day, Thomas Edison was considered more of an inventor—an applied scientist, not a pure, basic researcher. Nonetheless, Secretary of the Navy Josephus Daniels requested Edison's support to serve as the head of a new body of civilian experts, named the Naval Consulting

Board, to advise the navy on science and technology. One of the first initiatives planned by the Board was to create a modern research facility for the navy. In 1916, Congress allocated $1.5 million for the creation of the institution, but wartime delays and disagreements within the Naval Consulting Board postponed construction until 1920; the laboratory began operation in 1923 (NRL, 2001).

The laboratory's first projects included work on high-frequency radio and underwater sound propagation, improved communications equipment, and sonar. NRL produced the first practical radar equipment built in the United States. The laboratory moved gradually toward becoming a broadly based basic and applied research facility, and by World War II, five divisions had been added: Physical Optics, Chemistry, Metallurgy, Mechanics and Electricity, and Internal Communication. In 1941 NRL had a total of 396 employees and expenditures of close to $1.7 million. By 1946 the number of employees had reached 4,400 and expenditures close to $13.7 million; the number of buildings had increased from 23 to 67, and the number of projects from 200 to about 900. During World War II, scientific activities throughout the nation were concentrated almost entirely on applied research. NRL focused on developing and refining electronics equipment—radio, radar, and sonar. A thermal diffusion process was conceived and used to supply some of the U^{235} isotope needed for one of the first atomic bombs (NRL, 2001).

Because of scientific accomplishments during the war years, the United States sought to preserve the working relationship between its armed forces and the scientific community, desiring to consolidate its wartime gains in science and technology. The navy established the Office of Naval Research (ONR) as a liaison with and supporter of basic applied scientific research, and NRL was transferred to the administrative oversight of ONR, with a civilian director. At the same time, the laboratory's research emphasis shifted to one of long-range basic and applied investigation in a broad range of the physical sciences.

Since World War II, NRL programs in basic research have focused on the naval environments of earth, sea, sky, and space. Investigations include monitoring the sun's behavior, analyzing marine atmospheric conditions, and measuring parameters of the deep oceans. The laboratory also began naval research into space, becoming involved in such programs as the Vanguard project—America's first satellite program—the navy's Global Positioning System, and the Strategic Defense Initiative program. Recently, NRL was consolidated with the Naval Oceanographic and Atmospheric Research Laboratory to lead research in specialty areas of the ocean and atmospheric sciences (NRL, 2001).

1931: Lawrence Berkley Laboratory, U.S. High-Energy Particle Physics

The advent of high-energy particle physics can be traced to the turn of the nineteenth century and the study of nuclear physics, whose most notable scientists at that time were located in Europe. However, it was in the United States in 1930 that an American scientist by the name of Ernest Lawrence, an associate professor of physics at Berkeley, together with his graduate student M. Stanley Livingston, built the first successful "atom smasher" (called a cyclotron, or circular accelerator). The cyclotron became the primary tool that enabled scientists to study the components of the nucleus; several of Lawrence's original design components are still used in the accelerators built today. Lawrence and Livingston received a total of $1,000 in research funds from the university and NAS, which he used to build the million-volt cyclotron (Heilbron and Kevles, 1988). A few years later, during the Great Depression, Lawrence established the Radiation Lab ('Rad Lab'), the forerunner of the present Lawrence Berkeley Laboratory, with support from Berkeley, philanthropists, and the gift of an 80-ton magnet. With his accelerators, Lawrence committed his laboratory from 1934 until World War II to creating new radioisotopes with properties particularly adapted to biological research. Both the Rockefeller Foundation and the Macy Foundation encouraged Lawrence's attention to the creation of material for biomedical research. He received substantial sums from both philanthropies, and in turn created a supply of biologically active radioisotopes that included P^{32} and technetium (Heilbron et al., 1981).

In 1936, the University of California at Berkeley officially established the Radiation Laboratory as an independent entity within the Physics Department. The reorganized laboratory was dedicated to nuclear science rather than, as in its first incarnation, to accelerator physics. The focus on nuclear physics represented the hope that the potential sale of radioisotopes for biological research and medicine would support further cyclotron developments. Although a radiopharmaceutical industry did not materialize in the 1930s, the hope that it might do so helped sustain accelerator physics (Heilbron et al., 1981).

The focus, organization, and management of the Radiation Laboratory at Berkeley were soon to be altered by three important events, all occurring in 1939: World War II began; Ernest Lawrence won the Nobel Prize for his work on the cyclotron; and Niels Bohr, on a visit to the United States to attend a conference at the Carnegie Institution, announced to American scientists that two German scientists had discovered fission. These events would also have a permanent effect on the entire world of particle physics. Soon after the announcement on fission, laboratories around the world had duplicated the effect. The potential that fission—the splitting of an atom resulting in the release of a considerable amount of energy—could be used to create an enormous reactive explosion, created fear in the United States that German scientists might build a fission bomb (Goldberg, 1995). That same year Lawrence announced plans for a 100-megavolt cyclotron (Heilbron et al., 1981).

During 1940 a group of notable European scientists who had emigrated to the United States to escape the Nazi regime developed a technological program to explore the possibility of capitalizing on the energy released from nuclear fission. Private foundations were supporting research in nuclear physics, but no one was pursuing the potential explosive releases of fission energy. Spurred by the potential of Germany's progress in this area, immigrant scientists called upon their friend Albert Einstein to write and sign a letter informing President Roosevelt of the technological possibilities offered by fission. Five months later, Roosevelt responded by authorizing $6,000 to set up a committee on uranium research. Soon after, a crash program to build the first fission bomb, under the name of the Manhattan Project, began in the United States. The magnet for Lawrence's new 100–megavolt accelerator, completed as a wartime priority, helped in developing the machinery for making the first nuclear explosives (Goldberg, 1995).

By 1940 there were almost 23 cyclotrons in service, all financed by private patrons and states—not the federal government—and as is the case today, accelerators quickly outdated themselves. The wartime mobilization of the Radiation Laboratory brought irreversible changes in its size, scope, and corporate life. It became the embodiment of big science in physics. Its prewar development had provided a base on which the temporary expansion demanded by war could take place successfully. In 1940, Lawrence's proposal for a 100-megavolt accelerator was aggressive, costing over $1 million and requiring a corresponding increase in staff (Kevles, 1995). The award of the Nobel Prize in physics to Lawrence helped in his quest for money for the new machine among his usual sources. The Rockefeller Foundation pledged the principal amount of $1.4 million in April 1940, and OSRD contributed $400,000 in 1942 (Heilbron et al., 1981).

Most of the funds were used to purchase a cyclotron with a magnet face 184 inches in diameter. This magnet could not be housed on campus, and the laboratory was moved adjacent to the campus. The magnet was used to separate the explosive part of natural uranium, U^{235}, from the more plentiful companion isotope, U^{238}. Because of the technology design expertise housed in the Radiation Laboratory, General Leslie Groves contacted Berkeley in 1942, and requested that the laboratory design the huge electromagnetic complex that would be used to produce fissionable material and was to be constructed in Oak Ridge, Tennessee. Soon after, another substantial discovery was made at Berkeley when the Radiation Laboratory isolated plutonium. In 1943, emulating the uranium laboratory at Oak Ridge, General Groves began supervising the construction of a plant for plutonium production (Heilbron et al., 1981).

The war had mobilized all aspects of the Radiation Laboratory, from nuclear medicine to nuclear physics and chemistry. Discoveries had been made in examining the biological consequences of high-altitude flying. Using radioactive isotopes of inert gases, the cause of decompression sickness was discovered, and tracer studies at the laboratory made fundamental contributions to the understanding of the circulation and diffusion of gases. Other contributions in the form of practical devices, such as oxygen equipment, a parachute opener, and methods for measuring the rate of circulation and perfusion of the blood by capillaries, were also made by work done at the laboratory.

The surrender of Japan ended the emergency that had created the federally funded National Laboratories, but not the large organization and tight security that had come to characterize nuclear science. The methods and resources of big science, enlarged by the war, were to dominate the study of physics in peace as well. In February 1946, the Radiation Laboratory's semiannual budget, distributed by the army through the Manhattan Engineering District, amounted to $1,370,000 (Heilbron et al., 1981). As the war budget closed down, the Atomic Energy Commission (AEC, forerunner of the Department of Energy [DOE]), headed by a civilian commission under presidential control, took charge of the nuclear energy program in January 1947. The AEC formulated its research policy in 1947, with much input from the physicists at the National Laboratories, who advocated broad and strong support for basic scientific research. The newly organized AEC appropriated $15 million for the accelerators. Prohibited by the Atomic Energy Act of 1947 from giving grants for research, the agency developed a system of contracts with universities and established an independent Division of Research to administer them (Heilbron et al., 1981).

1937: The National Cancer Institute (NCI)

On August 5, 1937, President Roosevelt signed the National Cancer Institute Act into law. NCI was authorized to conduct and foster research and studies relating to methods of diagnosis and treatment of cancer; promote the coordination of cancer research; provide fellowships at the Institute; secure advice from cancer experts in the United States and abroad; and cooperate with state health agencies in the prevention, control, and eradication of cancer (Rettig, 1977). Included in this act was the establishment of an advisory body to NCI, the National Advisory Cancer

Council, authorized to review all research projects for approval. Funds were appropriated directly to NCI, not to the parent organization, NIH.

The organization of NCI occurred between the passage of the 1937 law and the entry of the United States into World War II. By 1939 the original research staff, consisting of 20 fellows recruited for their scientific competence, was settled in the new Institute building in Bethesda, Maryland. Through World War II, NCI's research program was conducted mainly in the Institute's own intramural laboratories, where organization was kept fluid, and scientific competence was the basis for establishing laboratory leadership (Rettig, 1977).

Not long after its organization, the scope of NCI's research program gradually developed beyond the intramural effort in its Bethesda laboratories to include extramural grants for clinical and basic research to university and medical school investigators. With an initial appropriation total of $500,000, the extramural program began slowly, those in charge calling the idea "unsound" (Rettig, 1977). In 1938, only 10 extramural grants totaling $90,000 were approved. During the war, funds remained limited, but in the two decades between 1937 and 1957, extramural expenditures totaled $45.2 million. NCI's clinical research program took off soon after the war with a clinical research center—the Laboratory of Experimental Oncology—being established jointly with the University of California San Francisco. In 1953, this clinical laboratory was closed, and NCI moved its clinical programs to the newly opened NIH Clinical Center on the Bethesda campus (Rettig, 1977).

NCI's program also funded state studies of cancer mortality and epidemiology, and provided advisory services to state health departments during World War II. This grant-in-aid program to the states had an annual program level that ranged from $2.2 to $3.5 million, with a total of $23.3 million spent from 1947 through 1957. The funds were used for cancer clinics, home nursing care, follow-up services, limited laboratory services for the indigent, statistical studies, and education (Rettig, 1977). NCI's extensive research program was used as a model by other NIH Institutes in establishing their own research programs.

Change in National Focus: Earth Sciences to Physical (Laboratory) Sciences

During the late nineteenth century, the years following the Civil War, federal support for research in the earth sciences had expanded enormously, supplying extraordinary investment to fields relevant to one of the major national missions of the era—the exploration, settlement, and economic development of the Far West. This increase in federally supported science displeased conservatives, who thought that the government was spending too much money for seemingly impractical work. The increase also upset populist-oriented congressmen, who did not see why funds should be spent for research on the things of the earth when human beings were earning too little to keep their farms. During the depression of the 1890s, these conservatives and reformers formed a coalition that sharply reduced the government's support for "impractical" science and forced bare-bones budgets on the federal scientific agencies (Kevles, 1995). Though the Depression was the occasion for the cutbacks, the geographical frontier had closed; the country was beginning to emphasize the agenda of its new urban industrial revolution, and the earth sciences agencies were no longer at the top of that agenda.

World War II

The efforts of the early American earth and biological scientists in the fields of geology, topography, paleontology, botany, and zoology had earned the respect of Europeans. In the 1870s, only about 75 Americans called themselves physicists, and almost all American physics was experimental rather than theoretical. In physics, chemistry, and astronomy, Americans had published only one-third as much work since the Revolution as their French and British colleagues (Kevles, 1995). At the turn of the twentieth century, using the momentum, experience, and scientific knowledge gained in the previous century's research activities, American science was poised to begin exploring new frontiers in the physical sciences. It took on new challenges during World War I, using research in the physical sciences to aid in the development and advancement of military technologies. By the advent of World War II, the government had already begun a pattern of investment in scientific research on which it would increasingly rely during the impending conflict.

1940–1941: National Defense Research Committee (NDRC) and Office of Scientific Research and Defense (OSRD)

Early in 1940, in light of "the upcoming conflict," President Franklin D. Roosevelt approved the organization of NDRC, which had been proposed by Vannevar Bush (president of Carnegie Institution of Washington, chair of the National Advisory Committee for Aeronautics [NACA], and ex-MIT vice president and dean of engineering). Financial support for NDRC was provided by presidential emergency funds authorized by Congress. Bush was appointed as chair of NDRC, which was organized to coordinate the scientific efforts in weaponry development of the government, the private sector, and universities. Bush used his experience as chair of NACA, an organization created by Congress to oversee and coordinate scientific study of the problems of flight, to establish similar mechanisms of research and development (R&D) management within NDRC. He continued and expanded his relatively novel use of the government contract system, greatly increasing the government's use of contracts for R&D services (facilities and expertise) that were available in the private and university sectors. NDRC delegated the responsibility for technical decisions concerning research to be pursued and managed at the institution level while maintaining a tight hold on the administration and coordination of the overall effort. NDRC made the revolutionary decision to ask universities to undertake war projects and brought American universities for the first time into large-scale research programs, ushering in a new period in the relationship between the federal government and institutions of higher education (Killian, 1982; Goldberg, 1995).

This approach required a new relationship among government, university, and the private sector, resulting in an infusion of public resources into university-based research. A year later (1941), at Bush's request, Roosevelt approved OSRD, an expansion and reorganization of government R&D activities, which included NDRC. OSRD expanded the development of agency-sponsored extramural research programs, entering into over 800 research contracts, mainly with universities, and expending in excess of $330,000,000 in completing these contracts. Under OSRD contracts, MIT began developing radar, Carnegie Institute of Technology (CIT) developed rockets, Harvard University worked on sonar, the University of Chicago worked on nuclear reactions, the University of California fabricated the first atomic bomb, and 69 academic institutions were represented on the staff of the Radiation Laboratory. Meanwhile, du Pont, General Electric, Union Carbide, and other industrial giants built the facilities to produce fissionable materials. Other contracts enabled the perfection of sulfa drugs and penicillin and the invention of insecticides, such as DDT (Killian, 1982; Price, 1962).

Vannevar Bush's contributions to the advancement of science and technology and the expansion of federal science policy in the United States have had a lasting impact. Although the official executive office of Scientific Advisor to the President was not organized until the Eisenhower Administration, Bush's influential involvement with Franklin Roosevelt during a critical period in the country's history and the wartime projects he organized had a significant effect on the course of American science.

1940–1945: The Manhattan Project

As noted above, certain events during World War II have had a considerable and lasting impact on federally funded, university-based scientific research. Arguably among the greatest contributors to the shift in large-scale government investment in university-based research was the Manhattan Project, which had a significant effect on the direction of federally funded basic research as we know it and gave rise to a new type of big-science project. At the time it was completed, the Manhattan Project could probably have claimed to be one of the largest government sponsors of university-based research.

In the United States prior to World War II, federal funds were available to a limited number of universities for scientific research. Physical science research activities at the turn of the century were small and purposely did not rely on expensive equipment, large expenditures, or many personnel. During the decade preceding the war, many advances in particle physics were made, sponsored in large part by private foundations. At the outset of the war, Vannevar Bush had jurisdiction within OSRD over investigations into the possibility of developing a nuclear bomb, the pursuit of which would rely heavily on promising advances in several fields of physics. Rumors that Germany was a year ahead in developing such technology spurred Bush to convene an NAS committee of chemists, physicists, and engineers, who were to answer the very narrow question of whether it would be feasible to use uranium to engineer a fission bomb. After three meetings over the course of 9 months, the panel reported that with sufficient effort over several years, success in doing so was a virtual certainty, and the effort would require $133 million (Goldberg, 1995). By 1941, work on uranium had proved very successful, and with the positive response from the NAS committee, Bush decided to make an immediate move. He reorganized the work on uranium, began designing production plants and reactors, and created three research centers to participate in the project—at Columbia University, the University of Chicago, and the Radiation Laboratory at Berkeley (Goldberg, 1995).

In June 1942, when the substantial costs required for production became obvious, Bush turned the project over to the Army Corps of Engineers, whose massive wartime budget could bury the effort, and where it could be disguised as the Manhattan Project. By October 1942, to speed up progress, Bush requested that Colonel Leslie R. Groves be appointed to lead the project. Groves' intention was to do whatever was required to build the bomb in the shortest amount of time and use it to end the war. It was Groves who, amid strong objections, appointed J. Robert Oppenheimer as director of a special new laboratory at Los Alamos that Groves set up specifically to design the bomb itself. Groves had the factories and plants built that were necessary to produce the fissionable materials and provided other services to the scientists as needs appeared. During the peak of the project in late 1944, over 160,000 people were employed in operations extending from coast to coast and in Canada as well (Heilbron et al., 1981; Goldberg, 1995). The bomb was completed in the summer of

1945, and by the end of World War II several weeks later, the original estimate of $133 million had grown to the $2 billion cost for the Manhattan Project ($20 billion in current dollars) (Goldberg, 1995). An incentive to build the bomb had been fear that Germany would do so first. Germany surrendered on May 7, 1945. On August 6 the United States dropped the first nuclear bomb on Hiroshima. The Russians declared war on Japan on August 8. On August 9 the United States dropped a second atomic bomb on Nagasaki. On August 14 the Japanese agreed to an unconditional surrender.

The field of high-energy physics grew at an incredible rate during the brief period of the war in those laboratories associated with designing the atomic bomb. Organization and management of these physics projects, conducted within the Manhattan Project, were directed largely by the federal government and in part by the scientist directors of individual research laboratories and facilities. Most of the research conducted by physicists, whether or not it was federally funded, was influenced and directed on some level by the federal government, and proceeded under tight security with the utmost secrecy. Despite this security and secrecy, however, most scientists believed that the pursuit of this science was not regimented. Scientists in both universities and industry were "free to make the most of the creative powers" (Killian, 1982). Many of the most notable physicists, several of whom were Nobel Laureates, became directors of the National Laboratories, including Los Alamos National Laboratory, the Radiation Laboratory at Berkeley, and the Fermi National Accelerator Laboratory. It was at these laboratories where many students were trained. Unfortunately, many graduate programs were put on hold during the war, but colleges and universities "had their dormitories and classrooms filled with Army and Navy trainees"(Killian, 1982). The training was necessary to staff the national and university research laboratories conducting research on novel war technologies such as sonar, radar, atomic and other weaponry, aircraft, optics, and antibiotics, to name a few.

The results of the Manhattan Project's investment in basic and applied research provide an obvious example of the essential role science plays as a prerequisite to technology development. These advances led to a continuation of the wartime policy of government support for university-based scientific research laboratories. The work on the atom bomb during the war raised a host of new questions, and officials in both the federal government and universities agreed that research in this area should have federal support, and should include funding for building the machines and for training undergraduate and graduate students. NDRC, OSRD, and the wartime federal contracts were destined to terminate with the end of the war. Many of those involved in these wartime efforts (with the interesting exception of most universities) believed that the new technological advances, the potential for more research developments, and the momentum gained in basic science research during the war should be maintained and even expanded after the war (Old, 1961). Toward the end of the war, various steps were taken to explore the possibility of a continued federal investment in public research efforts (Goldberg, 1995; Old, 1961).

Vannevar Bush was among those who wished federal investments in science to continue after the war. In response to a letter he had received from President Roosevelt inquiring about the returns from and economic value of this federal investment, Bush wrote a report entitled *Science: The Endless Frontier*. He stated: "We have no national policy for science. The Government has only begun to utilize science in the nation's welfare. There is no body within the Government charged with formulating or executing a national science policy. There are no standing committees in Congress devoted to this important subject. Science has been in the wings. It should be brought to the center of the stage—for in it lies much of our hope for the future" (Bush, 1945a).

Within the report, Bush outlined several notable and decisive achievements, but he carried his report beyond a response to Roosevelt's inquiries. His main emphasis was on the need for continued investment in scientific research and the development of a more refined and applicable science policy. He outlined the impact of science on the outcome of World War II. He emphasized that basic scientific research is scientific capital from which applied technologies are developed. The wealth of basic research before the war had aided in the development of radio, radar, penicillin, guided gunsites and bombsites, the atomic bomb (not mentioned in Bush's report, published in July 1945), and other technical developments that had been decisive in winning the war. Bush attributed these important advances to well-trained scientists and to the open and free environment that encouraged them to pursue basic science research. He mentioned that for many years, government had wisely supported research in the agricultural colleges, whose benefits had been great, and that this same system of support should be extended to other fields. He outlined the organization of a new federal agency with the sole purpose of supporting basic science research in the public domain. Bush's desire for such a science agency and the science policy he specifically outlined in his report was never fully realized. However, fragments of his ideas, along with the government's wartime investment in large-scale science research projects, did have an impact on the creation of a national science agency and on postwar science policy, influencing the precedents for current government involvement in science research.

Post-World War II

After the war, as the federal government worked on prioritizing its funding responsibilities, many agencies were created, and existing agencies were expanded. Several of the agencies that play key roles in funding current science research endeavors have their roots in this postwar period. The organization of new agencies facilitated the funding and coordination of both small- and large-scale science research projects in many different disciplines, and gave rise to both intramural and extramural research programs. The extramural grant system provided federal funding to universities for science research, but without interference from the government regarding the details of conducting individual research projects. The agencies discussed below have played major roles in continuing and expanding research activities within high-energy physics. Without the continuing support provided by these key agencies, research in this area would not have advanced as rapidly as it has.

Although domestic involvement has played a large part in the advancement of particle physics, soon after World War II it became apparent that success and efficiency in this field would depend upon international cooperation. Following the pattern established historically in the fields of astronomy, geology, and cartography in forming international communities, high-energy physics began, and has since sustained, large-scale international research collaborations.

1946: The Office of Naval Research (ONR)

As World War II unfolded, it became increasingly evident that the success of the Allied Forces could be attributed to the use of new technological advances in warfare. Many of these advances were developed by the scientists and engineers who had formerly been associated with university and industrial basic and applied research laboratories, but were assigned during the war to OSRD and NDRC. As these organizations were intended to terminate at the end of the war, a small group of naval reserve officers in the Office of the Secretary of the Navy began to consider how R&D should be organized within the Navy Department after the war. What worried these officers was that the Navy Department as organized in 1943 had no mechanism for liaison with key research scientists and engineers other than through OSRD. The basic question the naval officers addressed was how to enable the navy to establish and maintain relationships with top research scientists and engineers to continue the development of new weapons systems and operational capabilities. The naval reserve officers' group proposed a new office to oversee a novel organizational concept. This concept involved establishing, by an act of Congress, a special office under the secretary of the navy with its own budget and the authority to invest in and contract for basic and applied research (Old, 1961). The new office would be called the chief of naval research and could be held by a naval officer, but the office would require two safety valves. First, the chief of naval research must report to a civilian assistant secretary of the navy, who would be a recognized scientist or engineer capable of influencing a sound and rigorous R&D program. Second, a Naval Research Advisory Committee (NRAC), made up of nationally recognized leaders, would have to be formed to advise the secretary of the navy on research matters (Old, 1961).

This concept was completed by the end of 1943 and was promoted both inside the Navy Department and within the Executive Office of the President over the next 3 years. On August 1, 1946, the ONR was organized and received the $40 million the navy had in excess funds at the end of the war. ONR coordinated naval research, development, and test activities; managed activities relating to patents, inventions, trademarks, and copyrights; and sponsored many science and technology contracts in the postwar years. The achievements of university research during the war led the Department of Defense (DOD), through ONR, to generously fund on-campus basic research in the postwar period. ONR moved quickly to aid universities in reestablishing graduate programs in science and technology, setting a pattern of sponsorship that recognized the unique characteristics of universities—the essential values of academic freedom and the admission (and freedom of choice) of qualified students, including foreign nationals. ONR established contracting principles and procedures that paved the way for the National Science Foundation (NSF) and were generally adopted by all parts of DOD and by other government agencies, including the AEC (currently DOE) (Killian, 1982). ONR's charter was expanded from basic science to the management of all the navy's science and technology programs, and has played a major part in underwriting unclassified science and technology research (National Archives and Records Administration Records of the Office of Naval Research).

1946: The Department of Energy (DOE)

The origins of DOE can be traced to the Manhattan Project and the race to develop the atomic bomb during World War II. In 1942, the U.S. Army Corps of Engineers established the Manhattan Engineering District to manage the project. Following the war, Congress engaged in a vigorous and contentious debate over civilian versus military control of the atom. The Atomic Energy Act of 1946 settled the debate by creating the

AEC, which took over the Manhattan Engineering District's sprawling scientific and industrial complex.

The AEC was established specifically to maintain civilian government control over the field of atomic R&D. During the early years of the Cold War, it focused on designing and producing nuclear weapons and developing nuclear reactors for naval propulsion. The Atomic Energy Act of 1954 ended exclusive government use of the atom and initiated the growth of the commercial nuclear power industry, giving the AEC authority to regulate the new industry (U.S. Department of Energy, 2001).

In response to obvious conflicts of interest and disputes that mounted in the mid-1970s, the AEC was abolished, and the Energy Reorganization Act of 1974 created two new agencies. The Nuclear Regulatory Commission was organized to regulate the nuclear power industry, and the Energy Research and Development Administration was responsible for managing the nuclear weapon, naval reactor, and energy development programs (U.S. Department of Energy, 2001).

However, with the extended energy crisis of the 1970s came a need for unified energy organization and planning. The Department of Energy Organization Act brought the federal government's agencies and programs into a single agency. DOE, activated on October 1, 1977, assumed the responsibilities of the Federal Energy Administration, the Energy Research and Development Administration, the Federal Power Commission, and parts and programs of several other agencies.

Since its inception, DOE has shifted its focus as the needs of the nation have changed. During the late 1970s, it emphasized energy development and regulation. In the 1980s, nuclear weapons research, development, and production took priority. Since the end of the Cold War, DOE has focused on cleaning up the environment from the legacy of the Cold War, maintaining the safety and reliability of the U.S. nuclear stockpile, pursuing energy efficiency and conservation, developing innovations in science and technology, and fostering technology transfer and industrial competitiveness (U.S. Department of Energy, 2001).

1947: The National Laboratories (component of the DOE)

Several of the research centers created to support the Manhattan Project formed a set of "National Laboratories." These laboratories were incorporated into the AEC in 1947, which, as noted, later became DOE. As a result, accelerator physics (high-energy particle physics) became, and remains, a ward of the federal government. The National Laboratories are responsible for some of the largest government-sponsored collaborations in science. The size and expense of their machines make them unaffordable for any single university or state government. Currently there are several DOE-sponsored National Laboratories that carry out particle physics activities, including Brookhaven, Fermi, Thomas Jefferson, Oak Ridge, Sandia, Los Alamos, Argonne, and Lawrence Berkley National Laboratories.

1950: The National Science Foundation (NSF)

Directly after World War II, universities most commonly received contracts from specific agencies, such as DOD, the Department of Agriculture, or the Department of Commerce. In 1950, Congress, in response to the work of several national advisory committees, created NSF to provide scholarships and fellowships for advanced scientific education, and organized a competitive grants system that awarded large grants through university departments to individuals and teams of scientists.

1952: CERN—(European Organization for Nuclear Research)

Given the enormous and continually increasing costs associated with particle physics, it became apparent after World War II that success and the continued pursuit of knowledge in this field would depend on large-scale international collaborations. One of the first and most notable of such ventures was organized in 1952 as Conseil Europeen Pour La Rechierche Nucleaire (European Council for Nuclear Research). The word "Council" has since been replaced by "Organization," but the organization is still known by its original acronym, CERN. The enormous expense of building, maintaining, and operating the large particle conductors, colliders, and detectors was shared among several European nations that came together to design, finance, and construct the CERN facility. The establishment of CERN as an organization and as a facility encouraged the return of the European physicists who had emigrated to the United States as a result of World War II. CERN has had a unifying effect on the world of particle physics and operates for pure, basic research. The results of its experiments and theoretical work are available to the public. Scientists at CERN, attempting to design a tool to connect research collaborations and academic purposes throughout the world, created the World Wide Web (Galison and Hevly, 1992).

During the 1950s, in the midst of the Cold War, the success of CERN as a series of multinational collaborations spawned the idea of creating a world accelerator for world peace (Wilson, 1975). Many physicists believed that the pursuit of international science research projects would lessen the effects of the Cold War, and physicists worldwide, including scientists from the Soviet Union, gathered for conferences to discuss collaborations. The well-known Rochester Conferences brought particle physicists together from around the world in an attempt to reopen scientific communication after the first icy decade of the Cold War. In 1957, the International Union of Pure and Applied Physics (IUPAP) was established to "encourage international collaboration among the various high-energy laboratories to ensure the best use of the facilities of these large and expensive installations" (Wilson, 1975).

1954: The President's Science Advisor

The evolution of the office of science advisor to the President was likely influenced by several factors, including Vannevar Bush's key role in World War II, his famous report *Science: The Endless Frontier*, and William T. Golden's report to President Truman recommending the creation of the position. These reports, along with the Soviet Union's successful Sputnik program, motivated President Eisenhower to elevate the status of his scientific advisors by creating the President's Science Advisory Committee (PSAC) and naming James R. Killian, president of MIT, as his full-time science advisor. Killian's introduction of a group of distinguished scientists into the government process to expand the level of scientific advice offered directly to the President began the tradition of having scientists contribute regularly to the formation of U.S. scientific policy (Kolb and Hoddeson, 1992). Although the office of science advisor to the President and PSAC were abolished by President Nixon in 1972, the advisory role was later expanded and reorganized in the National Science and Technology Policy, Organization, and Priorities Act of 1976 (Public Law 94-282), which established the Executive Office of Science Technology Policy (OSTP) that exists today (Dupree, 1986; Kolb and Hoddeson, 1992; OSTP, 2001).

1989: The End of the Cold War

The momentum gained in facilities, research, and training as a result of the Manhattan Project and the new government policy measures to support basic science research at universities gave American high-energy physicists a great head start after the war. This momentum continued and increased as a result of the Cold War. The hostility between the Soviet Union and the West compelled the United States to retain its preeminence in particle physics by funding the building of large facilities as academic laboratories to train new physicists and engineers who were needed to staff the National Laboratories.

In the midst of the Cold War, the field of physics experienced a shifting of national priorities similar to that faced by the earth sciences a century before. Similar to the coalition formed in the late 1800s to deter legislators from providing the accustomed funds for earth science research, a coalition formed in the 1960s believed that physics was too great an absorber of tax dollars, not attentive enough to social issues, and too much a creature of the military and the war in Vietnam. An attack on big science started in 1964 with the free speech movement on the Berkeley campus of the University of California, where science was seen as the demonic force that had produced the hydrogen bomb (Dupree, 1986). It was this coalition that forced a leveling of the growth of federal funds for physics. This shift had much more far-reaching effects than the cutbacks of the 1890s, when federal patronage of science had been largely confined to support for work carried out directly by federal agencies. By the mid-1970s, the federal budget for R&D was 20 percent lower in constant dollars than it had been in 1967, but the number of physicists was higher (Kevles, 1995). Despite the constant dollar fluctuations, particle physics did receive continued funding during the Cold War. However, the landscape for high-energy physics changed rather abruptly with the conclusion of the Cold War, and funding levels in the physical sciences are currently 20 percent lower than they were in the mid-1980s (NRC, 2001).

1787	Constitutional Convention
1789	Organization of the government
1790	First patent law; first census
1792	The Mint
1798	Medical care for merchant seamen
1800	Library of Congress
1802	Army Corps of Engineers; United States Military Academy, West Point, New York
1803	Lewis and Clark expedition
1807	Coast Survey Act
1813	Federal law establishing vaccine agent
1819	Long expedition to the Rockies
1830	Navy Depot of Charts and Instruments
1836	Reorganization of Patent Office
1838	United States Exploring Expedition
1840	National Institute for the Promotion of Science
1842	Naval Observatory; United States Botanical Garden
1845	United States Naval Academy
1846	Smithsonian Institute
1848	American Association for the Advancement of Science (AAAS)

1849   Bache's presidential address before AAAS
1850   President Buchanan's veto of land-grant college bill
1861   Government Printing Office; Outbreak of the Civil War
1862   Department of Agriculture; Homestead Act; Morrill Act for land-grant
        colleges
1863   National Academy of Sciences; Army Signal Corps
1866   Navy Hydrographic Office separated from Naval Observatory
1867   King's geological survey of fortieth parallel
1869   Wheeler's geographical surveys west of hundredth meridian
1870   Meteorological work begins in Army Signal Corps; Powell's
        geographical survey of Colorado River
1873   Hayden's geological/geographical survey of the territories
1879   U.S. Geological Survey; National Board on Health
1881   Founding of *Science* journal
1887   Hygienic Laboratory; Hatch Act for Agricultural Experiment Stations
1890   Transfer of meteorological service from Army to Department of
        Agriculture, creating the National Weather Bureau
1891   Astrophysical Observatory at Smithsonian Institute
1893   Army Medical School
1901   National Bureau of Standards; Bureaus of Chemistry, Plant Industry,
        and Soils in Department of Agriculture
1903   Committee on Organization of Scientific Work
1906   Pure Food and Drug Act
1912   Public Health Service
1915   National Advisory Committee on Aeronautics; Naval
        Consulting Board
1916   National Research Council; National Park Service
1917   Entry into World War I
1918   Chemical Warfare Service
1923   Naval Research Laboratory
1926   National Research Fund
1930   National Institute of Health
1933   Science Advisory Board
1937   National Cancer Institute
1938   *Research: A National Resource*
1940   National Defense Research Committee
1941   Office of Scientific Research and Development; entry into World War II
1946   Atomic Energy Commission; Office of Naval Research
1950   National Science Foundation
1954   Creation of President's Science Advisor

FIGURE A-1   Chronology of government-funded science.
SOURCE: Dupree, 1986: 383–86.

PART II: ISSUES IN CONDUCTING LARGE SCALE
COLLABORATIONS IN HIGH-ENERGY PARTICLE PHYSICS

In 1967, Alvin Weinberg, Director of Research at Oak Ridge National Laboratory, wrote in reference to his term "big science" that "many of the activities of modern science—nuclear physics, or elementary particle physics, or space research—require extremely elaborate equipment and staffs of large teams of professionals" (Weinberg, 1967). Weinberg continued by noting a series of conflicts and problems created by the emergence of big science, including the need to establish criteria for allocation of resources; to mediate among the interests of competing laboratories and individuals; and to provide for equitable distribution of funds (and as a result talent) between large-scale and small projects, as well as among different regions of the country. Since Weinberg first called explicit attention to big science, the phenomenon and the resulting difficulties have only increased and intensified. The results of some of the larger physics projects now being pursued are reported in papers listing hundreds of individual coauthors. The funding of the Human Genome Project, the dissolution of the Superconducting Super Collider, research on AIDS and cancer, and the hotly debated fiscal year 2002 science appropriations are some of the better-known examples of the current tensions in our society over the question of the proper niche for the social institutions of science (Goldberg, 1995).

Alvin Weinberg coined the phrase "big science" and some of the issues associated with it in 1961. Since then, many fields have made claims to pursuing 'big science' projects. The following section discusses some of the issues associated with large-scale research projects in particle physics. The term large-scale, in the following section, is loosely defined to include projects that are multi-institutional collaborations over a long period of time (5+ years), and receive multi-million dollar funds each year, directed primarily toward building and maintaining advanced-technology research facilities. Surprisingly, after 40 years of bigger and more expensive science, the issues of how best to prioritize, fund, organize, manage, and staff large projects and train students involved in these projects remain in many fields that conduct large-scale research projects.

In an attempt to understand and pinpoint specific issues associated with big science, the American Institute of Physics (AIP) conducted a three-phase *Study of Multi-Institutional Collaborations*, phase I of which was devoted entirely to the field of high-energy particle physics. Studying trends in collaborations in particle physics essentially means studying trends within the field itself. The majority, if not all, of significant projects in particle physics involve a multi-institutional collaboration. Within the

AIP study, the expectation was that each specialty would have particular traditions and needs that would shape the character of its collaborations. In other words, AIP expected to discern some sort of pattern in the conduct of large-scale projects. According to the AIP study, however, "we searched for a characteristic pattern within each specialty; we rarely found one. Instead, we found significant variations in collaborations within each field. Subsequent analysis of a database covering all three phases of the AIP Study bore out the conclusion that discipline-specific styles of multi-institutional collaborations do not exist" (1992).

The following discussion relies to the extent possible on information available specifically for the field of particle physics, but when necessary draws on information available from the general and broad field of physics, as described by government agencies and policy makers. The discussion is largely a summary of AIP's relevant survey findings regarding such large-scale research issues as funding, organization, management, staffing and training, and intellectual property, with some related information gathered from other sources. It should be noted that there is significant overlap among many of these issues, and this overlap is reflected in the discussion here.

Funding

Within the U.S. democratic system, the process of appropriating federal funds has been, and will most likely continue to be, highly complex. Determining funding priorities in a fluctuating social and economic environment is bound to leave some happier than others. A major issue the United States government faces in relation to its science and technology effort is how much money to allocate to science and technology as a whole, and how to divide that money among the various claimants in the science and technology community (Green, 1995). Even within a discipline, the distribution of funds can be contentious, as demonstrated in the 1995 National Research Council report *Setting Priorities for Space Research: An Experiment in Methodology*, in which there is no consensus on how to make these allocations. Several specific funding issues are associated with big-science projects, including the government's general allocations to a particular field, the specific allocations within a field between large and small projects, and the allocation of funds between basic and applied research programs.

Allocation of Federal Science Research Funds

The process of allocating federal funds in the United States is much more complex and detailed than the following summary (see Figure 4.1).

Simplified, the process begins when the President writes and submits a detailed budget that includes many line-item requests about 15 months prior to the start of the budget's fiscal year. The President's budget is submitted to Congress, to both the House and Senate budget committees. The two budget committees review and make changes to broad funding areas, called functions, in the areas of health, defense, civilian R&D, and so on. Congressional authorizing committees may then authorize or not authorize (as it did when it came close to not authorizing funds for the space station) the use of the funds for specific government agencies and programs. The revised budget is next given to the House and Senate full appropriations committees and is divided among the 13 corresponding appropriation subcommittees, which are mirrored on the House and Senate side (see Table 4.1). Although specific budget items may have been outlined by the President, the budget committees, and the authorizing committees, the appropriations committees also have some say in the amount of funds distributed to each of the agencies that falls under their jurisdiction. (In 1994, for example, the VA, HUD, and Independent Agencies appropriations conference committee chose not to appropriate funds to the Office of Technology Assessment, and essentially terminating that agency.) At this stage, several different agency budgets could be in competition for the funds available under the jurisdiction of an individual appropriations committee. Each of the 13 appropriations subcommittees from the House and Senate writes a bill that is submitted back to the respective full committee. The bills are taken to the House or Senate floor. Once approved, they next move to a congressional conference committee made up of House and Senate members from the corresponding appropriations subcommittees. The further-revised budget, a compromise of sorts between the House and Senate made up of 13 individual bills, is taken back to the floor and voted on. If approved, the bills (budget) go back to the President. When the President signs the final budget, it becomes law (U.S. Congressional Yellow Book, 2001).

The priorities set by the government and used to distribute the limited funds are determined by a variety of issues that usually reflect the most pressing needs of the nation, such as the state of domestic or foreign affairs and national security. Within the individual science funding agencies and the specific disciplines, mechanisms in place that help in setting priorities include the individual agency advisory committees, peer review mechanisms, the Office of Science and Technology Policy and various other White House advisory committees, and the National Research Council system. Even with these mechanisms in place, however, there is no avoiding competition among the various claims on federal funds, and there is no policy in place for what to do when there is just not enough money to go around—when the political system decides it has other priorities. According to former Representative Bill Green (New York), "We are, after all, dealing with a perfectly normal situation in which the useful things on which we can spend money require more money than we have to spend" (Green, 1995).

Traditional University Funding Mechanism

Continuing a practice that dates back to World War II, university physics departments have traditionally administered the federal research funds they receive for their high-energy physicists. This process makes it difficult to calculate and compare the cost of individual experiments because the university's contributions are embedded in all other high-energy physics activities. The benefits of this system have been the stability of universities relative to transitory collaboration groups and the university regulation of individual faculty activities (American Institute of Physics, 1992). This approach has also encouraged multi-institutional and international collaborations; a group with the ambition to build an expensive experiment must convince physicists from other institutions or countries to contribute support. An interesting find of the AIP survey was that most academic physicists expected their contracts with the funding agencies to cover travel and the operation of university laboratories and facilities, and to support postdoctoral and graduate students. The funds they were most concerned about acquiring were for the expensive materials and services needed to construct major new detector components (American Institute of Physics, 1992).

The larger, more recent collider experiments have not followed this tradition. In these cases, the government has provided the large accelerator laboratories with funds for detector development, and the laboratories have distributed the money among the collaborations with approved experiments. This laboratory-centered approach to funding experiments appears to be part of a trend to make the laboratories responsible for overseeing the collaborations that perform large, expensive experiments (AIP, 1992).

Large-Scale Versus Small-Scale Research

The debate over whether to fund large or small projects in the field of high-energy particle physics is somewhat moot because the expense associated with pursuing research in this area has mandated ever-larger collaborations that are almost always considered big science. It was reported within the AIP survey that one high-energy physicist had actually left the field so as not to have to work in a large collaboration.

The concern about smaller science projects losing funds to big science has been voiced in other fields. In the wake of the Human Genome Project, many life scientists, expressed a fear of "centralized control, bureaucracy and political considerations inevitable in big science, and the possibility that major appropriations for a large project in biology would diminish the funds available for small-scale activities in other fields of biological research" (Heilbron and Kevles, 1988). These concerns are voiced primarily by scientists who associate big science with an applied research approach and smaller projects with basic research. These scientists fear that funds will increasingly be directed toward applied science, inevitably decreasing the funds available for essential basic science research (King, 1991). (See the discussion in the next section.) Scientists have also expressed concern that funding large-scale research rather than small projects will result in a loss of research independence to more directed research projects. These concerns are not as great among high-energy particle physicists because most of the experiments conducted at accelerators are attempting to explore unknown frontiers and answer fundamental questions, and research pursuits are seldom directed by the facilities.

Basic Versus Applied Research

Several noteworthy scientists have emphasized the importance of always maintaining a solid basic science research program (Bush, 1945b; Price, 1962; Smith, 1998). Vannevar Bush stressed the necessity of pursuing such research to ensure a supply of solutions for present and future problems (1945b). He believed this type of research was best suited for an academic setting, but that it should be funded by the government. He also believed that while universities had the responsibility of pursuing this basic research, government and industry were responsible for translating its results into applied technologies. The system has developed much differently, however, with all three institutions involved in an evolving overlap of both types of research.

The importance of basic research in high-energy particle physics can be demonstrated by the devices and techniques resulting from fundamental research projects. According to a recent National Research Council report on the current state of physics:

> [It is] widely recognized that the federal government should take primary responsibility for the support of basic research in science, research that is vital for the needs of our nation. Such research is often too broad and distant from commercial development to be a sensible industrial investment. This is particularly true for physics. As a fundamental science, it tends to have a long time lag between discovery in the research lab and impact on the lives of citizens, but by the same token its impact can be all the more profound. Ten to twenty years is a typical interval between a fundamental physics discovery and its impact on society. This

can be seen with the laser, magnetic resonance imaging, the optical-fiber transmission line, and many other examples. Much of today's high-tech economy is being driven by the technology that grew out of physics research in the early 1980's. (National Research Council, 2001).

Other contributions, along with various medical imaging technologies, include developments in cancer therapy; radiation processing; food, medical, and sewage sterilization; national security technology; and the World Wide Web, developed at CERN (Smith, 1998). These developments are positive examples of the law of unintended consequences (Groopman, 2001).

Organization

Most of the large collaborations in high-energy physics are organized before a proposal has been written and submitted to the accelerator laboratory. In general, a proposal is written after the collaboration has been organized, and is produced by a group of scientists who have, or are building, a detector. The proposal is submitted to the accelerator laboratory; if it is approved, the collaboration will be able to use its detector at the laboratory facility. Organizers of experiments need to attract enough physicists to an experiment to convince the large accelerator laboratory administrators that the experiment, if approved, could be built and run as proposed. These large accelerator facilities require detailed contracts called Memoranda of Understanding (MOUs), covering the responsibilities of both the laboratory and each of the institutional members of the collaboration performing the experiments. This relatively new requirement is indicative of the current trend in the shifts of power and accountability mentioned above in the section on funding (American Institute of Physics, 1992).

The responsibilities of an experiment organizer vary depending upon the specific experiment(s), but in general, all organizers must determine the size of the consortium, choose the collaborators, organize experiment strategies, and ensure appropriate communication. International collaborations have become almost the norm in high-energy physics experiments and generate a unique set of issues, as discussed below.

Size and Personnel

The need for additional, larger, and increasingly sophisticated instruments has increased the number of physicists a potential experiment organizer must mobilize, while at the same time competition for the field's funds and personnel has been a factor in keeping collaborations lean in relation to the tasks undertaken. As a result, experiment organizers tend to worry about gathering enough collaborators for an experiment. They do not, however, according to the AIP survey, worry about compiling a complementary blend of skills and subspecialties. They assume that individual American physicists are familiar with, if not expert in, all phases of an experiment, and that a university group has all the skills needed for an experiment, with graduate students participating in the full range of work as part of their training (American Institute of Physics, 1992). Interestingly, other scientists participating in the survey expressed contradictory sentiments regarding current graduate education, expressing concern that large projects were limiting the breadth of education students received, constraining their participation to isolated segments of the experiments.

Because academic particle physicists in the United States are funded as university groups with limited resources, and the accelerator laboratory groups are few in number, collaborations become larger only by including more domestic academic institutions or foreign groups. The addition of institutions does bring collaborations the needed additional resources, but also increases organizational complexity. This fundamental trade-off between increased resources and collaboration complexity, accompanied by the inevitable internal competition, has probably been the greatest source of daily friction within the large collaborations (American Institute of Physics, 1992).

Choosing Collaborators

Most of the collaborations in high-energy physics form to take advantage of a new accelerator facility or component, for detector construction, for data analysis, or for computer programming. AIP's survey found no formula that organizers could use for choosing compatible collaborators, though logistical convenience, the availability of appropriate personnel, and technical expertise were primary factors in producing a collaboration for building a detector. Preexisting professional relationships and personal contacts played a significant role as well. Would-be experiment organizers have also used summer programs and open meetings to enlarge their circle of colleagues. Other collaborations have been formed when large accelerator facilities combined separate teams of scientists who had submitted similar research proposals into "shotgun marriages." One element cited as key in forming a workable collaboration was the ability of experimenters to work harmoniously with the accelerator laboratory's staff. Scientists concur that they have better relations with laboratory staff by including physicists from the laboratory's research division in the collaboration. Most university-based experiment organizers surveyed had consciously tried to include accelerator physicists as collaborators (American Institute of Physics, 1992).

Despite an organizer's best efforts, AIP concluded that characteristics of the available instrumentation can constrain the social and organizational options physicists confront in collaborative research. It was also found that collaborations are relatively less productive compared with the small facilities at universities and the small research groups that operate the accelerator laboratories. This lower productivity can limit the short- or long-term willingness of physicists to work together in particular collaborations (American Institute of Physics, 1992).

Communication

Intracollaboration communications have become increasingly formal (collaboration-wide mailings and memoranda) and increasingly electronic in the larger, more recent experiments. Even though organizers of collaborations try to keep them as small as possible, the larger collaborations have created administrative positions and subgroups to deal with matters that were handled collectively or by individuals in smaller collaborations. For large and small groups, the collaboration meetings have remained the key communication mechanism used by physicists to discuss decisions concerning the tactics and results of experiments. Even scientists who found such meetings unpleasant did not suggest alternatives to their use as the preferred way of debating and resolving the physics issues involved in an experiment (American Institute of Physics, 1992).

International Collaborations

International collaborations have increasingly become necessary to make experiments feasible. Reasons for forming these consortia include the desire to use and learn an experimental technique developed by a foreign group, the need of a domestic experiment for more manpower and money, a brokered merger by a facility director between domestic and foreign collaborators who had submitted similar proposals, and the desire of U.S. scientists with a working detector for more beam time than a U.S. accelerator would provide. These collaborations have experienced several problems beyond the language barrier, including technical, cultural, logistical, and political-legal issues (American Institute of Physics, 1992).

Management

Management of a high-energy physics collaboration may include such matters as designing, building, maintaining, adjusting, and running accelerators and detectors, and determining the priority of experiments to be conducted. The national accelerator laboratories have always been responsible for supporting university research (by providing "beam time"), as well as their own research groups. Traditionally, interuniversity collaborations have been formed to provide enough physicists to build and run experiments to ensure that a proposal would be approved and funded by an accelerator facility. The collaborators would design and build the detector at their home institutions without oversight from the national laboratories. Over the past few decades, as experiments have increased in size and expense and as the quality of university laboratories and shop facilities has declined, there has been an increase in the fabrication of detector components at the accelerator sites, resulting in tighter control over the experiments by the national laboratory facilities. As a result, funding is increasingly likely to come directly to the government laboratories for distribution to the collaboration groups. Most collaborations must choose a manager (known as the spokesperson) from their staff who may be required to remain on site for the duration of the experiment, and collaborations must also submit an MOU detailing the responsibilities of consortium members in relation to the experiments. The loss of a collaboration's administrative autonomy to large facilities, in conjunction with the dependence on using the instrumentation provided by the facilities that is crucial to high-energy physics, has affected all phases of collaborative research (American Institute of Physics, 1992).

The Spokesperson

The spokesperson is an individual designated as a liaison between the collaboration and the accelerator facility. Spokespersons usually familiarize themselves with all aspects of the experiments. Although the spokesperson is posed as an administrative role, collaborations usually make the experiment's instigator their spokesperson, and the role carries connotations of scientific initiative and leadership. Because of the diminished powers to reward and discipline members of a collaboration, spokespersons reason and persuade their way through conflicts and misunderstandings, and retention of their position is treated as evidence of leadership and scientific judgment. Junior faculty on experiments desire the office of spokesperson in the belief that it will help their tenure campaigns (American Institute of Physics, 1992).

Management Issues

Collaboration dynamics raise several problems cited by the AIP survey respondents. The following were the problems most commonly noted:

when a narrowly focused experiment involved more faculty than it had physics topics to address, it was prone to divisive disputes over credit for the results obtained; when a physicist could use a detector to address multiple topics but only one topic at a time, other faculty would usually adopt one of the possible lines of inquiry and then fight over whose interests deserved collaboration-wide support; and when a productive but aging detector needed an upgrade, it became difficult to regulate competition within the collaboration for building a new component. In all these situations, unilateral actions or perpetual debate could preempt collective decision making (American Institute of Physics, 1992).

In April 2001, the National Research Council released its physics survey findings in a report entitled *Physics in a New Era: An Overview*. In conjunction with the release of that report, NRC sponsored a public webcast where it presented and discussed the survey findings and the report's recommendations. A major recommendation addressed the need for greater emphasis on appropriate training at all levels in physics education, from elementary education through postdoctoral training. During the question-and-answer segment following the summary of findings and recommendations, a question was posed about the recommendations made concerning physics education. The question specifically asked whether the committee had addressed the obvious need to train physicists to manage all the complexities involved in large-scale research projects. The committee spokesperson responded by saying this had been recognized as an issue, but the committee had not addressed it in detail, suggesting in the report the use of joint programs between business schools and physics departments. Although large-scale physics projects have been around for decades with the same issues, the problem of how to train scientists to manage these complex collaborations persists.

Compensation, Career Advancement, and Academic Recognition

According to AIP (1992), "The collaborations in our sample lacked the administrative powers to reward and discipline their faculty-level members. Promotions, pay raises, hiring privileges, the administration of research grants, and access to a machine shop or research and development laboratory all rested with the several institutions that employed the collaborators." Other constraints besides a lack of administrative authority may inhibit career progression. According to a former Fermilab director, the growth of big science is shrinking the job market. "We get fewer scientists per dollar" because more money is going into the construction of massive experimental apparatuses, and less into salaries (Flam, 1992). Along with the issue of low salaries is that of receiving credit for contributions to experiments. Journal papers in high-energy physics can sometimes have hundreds of authors. Even with smaller publications, collaborations attempting to recognize an individual's contributions by placing that individual's name at the head of the author list for the paper invariably provoke contention, especially when students are vying for the distinction. AIP suggests that collaborations should probably abandon this practice, especially with students, because word of mouth, letters of recommendation, and participation in conferences can effectively build reputations within the high-energy physics community (American Institute of Physics, 1992). This recommendation may be appropriate for the field of high-energy particle physics because of its relatively small size and the common practice of large collaborations. It would not be feasible within biomedical science as the number of scientists is several times that found in particle physics, and the research is most often practiced on a much smaller scale.

According to the AIP survey, to help graduate students and junior faculty gain recognition, a collaboration would carefully distribute conference talks to confer credit and provide exposure to the collaboration's lesser-known members. Managers and organizers who were "more enlightened and self-secure" would grant leadership opportunities to more junior people with the inspiration and ambition to organize and run an experiment within a collaboration. The most desired role of junior faculty was the office of spokesperson, which, as noted, was believed to be a great advantage for gaining tenure (American Institute of Physics, 1992).

Finally, despite the above-noted report of a physicist leaving the field of high-energy physics rather than working in ever-expanding collaborations, many scientists on the inside indicated in the AIP survey that they had found satisfaction in large collaborations even when they had expected to feel uncomfortable (American Institute of Physics, 1992).

Universities Research Association (URA), Inc.

President Lyndon Johnson's Science Advisory Committee and the National Academy of Sciences initiated the not-for-profit URA Corporation in 1965 for "the management and operation of research facilities in the national interest." These laboratories have traditionally been associated with expensive large-scale physics projects conducted at accelerator facilities. Specifically, URA was organized to create the Fermi National Accelerator Laboratory (Fermilab). Since January 1967, URA has been the prime contractor to DOE for the design, building, and operation of Fermilab, which houses the Tevatron, currently the world's highest-energy accelerator for elementary particle physics research. Presidents of participating universities designate their scientific and administrative talent to participate within the URA governing structure. URA is a consortium of 89 leading universities located primarily in the United States (including Cornell, Caltech, Berkeley, Stanford, Harvard, Yale, and MIT), with members also in Canada, Japan, and Italy.

URA's charter is ". . . to acquire, plan, construct, and operate machines, laboratories, and other facilities, under contract with the Government of the United States or otherwise, for research, development and education in the physical and biological sciences . . . and to educate and train technical, research and student personnel in said sciences" (URA, 2001). The corporation acts under the authority of its governing body, the Council of Presidents of its 89 member universities. A board of trustees appoints boards of overseers for each major research activity. URA's headquarters in Washington, D.C., coordinates the activities of the council and boards. URA's most notable responsibility is for oversight and governance of Fermilab and for corporate relations with the Federal Government, industry, academe, and the general public in matters of physics.

For fiscal year 2001, DOE funding for URA's contracts was approximately $289 million, National Science Foundation (NSF) funding was about $2 million, and National Aeronautics and Space Administration (NASA) funding was about $2 million (URA, 2001).

Staffing and Training

With a national policy for publicly funded science research having been developed only decades ago (Bush, 1945a), it is not surprising that career trends and associated issues in the field of high-energy particle physics have paralleled, with a small time lag, the availability of federal funding (see Figures A-2 and A-3). There is no policy in place to ameliorate the effects of shifting federal funds on programs and personnel involved in government-supported science research. In the words of Bozeman (1995), many scientists "have been the victims of social and political forces over which they have no control." Described below are several events involving government decisions and their effects on the projects, training, and careers of physicists. It is difficult to isolate one particular issue from others, and just as difficult to trace specific effects to specific causes. Thus, the events outlined below have also most likely influenced the funding levels, management, and organization of large science research projects, and the discussion here may note aspects of these other areas as well. As with many decisions, there is a lag time between when a decision is made, and when its effects become apparent; this is true for fiscal budget decisions, making it difficult to predict and manage the effects of federal funding decisions.

Government investment in large-scale university physics research

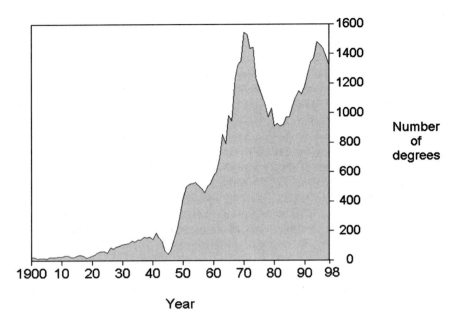

FIGURE A-2   Number of physics Ph.D.s conferred in the United States, 1900–1998.
SOURCE: NRC (2001).

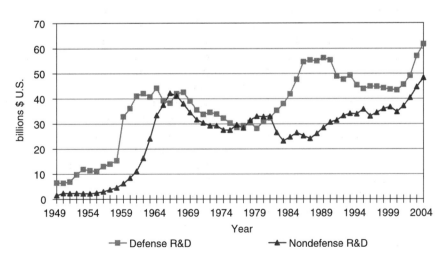

FIGURE A-3   Federal spending on defense and nondefense R&D: outlays for the conduct of R&D, FY 1949–2004, billions of constant FY 2003 dollars.
SOURCE: AAAS (2003).

during World War II, leading to immense expenditures in this area, had several significant results. Along with the development of sizeable and high-quality research facilities, these results include the extensive use of the federal contract system to fund sustained university research, the introduction of the scientist managers appointed to principal management roles in large-scale research projects, the involvement of notable scientists in government policy making, the creation of new and larger graduate programs, and the training of university undergraduate and graduate students.

Growth in physics continued after World War II with the onset of the Cold War. The hostility between the Soviet Union and the West compelled the United States to retain its preeminence in particle physics by funding the building of large facilities as academic laboratories to train new physicists and engineers who were needed to staff the national laboratories. National and international competition within the field and a concern to fill the demand for a "supply of well-trained physicists, engineers, and technicians produced Nobel prizes, national prestige, substantive knowledge, and many persons with doctorates in science and engineering" (Heilbron and Kevles, 1988).

In the midst of the Cold War, however, opposition was voiced that physics had become too large and expensive, provided little of social consequence, and was too closely associated with the military (in support of the Vietnam War). As mentioned above, this opposition resulted in a leveling in the growth of federal funds for physics. Although the federal budget (in constant dollars) for R&D had dropped 20 percent by the mid-1970s, the number of physicists had increased. Since the federal government was the primary supporter of basic physics research everywhere it was practiced, the contraction in funding adversely affected virtually the entire enterprise of the physical sciences in the United States, making jobs in academic physics, the center of basic research in many areas of the subject, particularly difficult to find. High-energy accelerators were shut down, and many research programs were terminated (Kevles, 1995). During this same time, accelerator facilities were becoming outdated, and the beginning of an energy crisis was making these facilities too expensive to maintain. As the smaller university facilities closed, a select few of the larger, more sophisticated, and efficient facilities were becoming centers of collaborative research. During the early 1980s, funding for physics research rose again, but the increase was short-lived after the Cold War ended in 1989.

The dependence on government funding for university-based research and training caused several problems after the Cold War in the early 1990s. The loss of the Superconducting Super Collider in 1993 drew a rather dramatic response from high-energy physicists, who feared it would mark the death of their field (Flam, 1992). As funding waned, headlines appeared such as "Physics Famine: A Frenzied Search for Job Stability," "Taking Roads Less Traveled by Researchers: Ph.D's Are Striking Off into Areas Such as Business and High School Teaching, With Mixed Success," and "Unemployment Blues: A Report from the Field" (Flam, 1992; Chollar, 1994; Tobias, 1994). Nobelist Leon Lederman stated, "Industry is shucking research, universities are retrenching, and national labs are on a decayed mission and don't know what they are going to do" (Flam, 1992). The relatively steady federal investment in physics research after World War II and through the Cold War era had created large training programs, numerous research projects, and a plethora of physicists. The decrease in physics funding after the Cold War, compounded by an influx of foreign students and scientists (see Figure A-4), left many physicists at every stage of the traditional career path without clear prospects.

Throughout the 1990s, the landscape for many physicists was unpredictable. Trained physicists had to find employment outside of traditional channels. AIP conducted several surveys and found physicists employed in all kinds of businesses, from venture capital, to finance, to running their own companies (Chollar, 1994). They became teachers, engineers, computer scientists, or consultants. Many students felt misled, believing that they had not been properly informed by their mentors about the lack of jobs and funding within the field. A large population of newly trained physicists with fewer traditional career options caused physics graduate training programs to come under scrutiny. Within the field there was a contradiction with regard to graduate training expectations. Most physicist mentors expected their graduate students to participate in all types of work, including the design, construction, running, and analysis of an experiment, as part of their training (American Institute of Physics, 1992). For most mentors, this expectation paralleled the training they had received, but they had undergone that training on significantly smaller, shorter, and less complex experiments. Other individuals lamented the effect of the length and complexity of experiments on graduate education, believing that long construction times were interfering with students' ability to both build the hardware and analyze data from the same experiment. The current system encourages a student to either develop the technical expertise necessary to keep an experiment going or analyze data from a previous experiment. It forces students to spend too much time on too few stages. To alleviate this situation, some scientists have recommended that graduate students analyze data from an experiment already under way while designing and building an apparatus to be used after receiving their degrees (American Institute of Physics, 1992).

Toward the latter part of the 1990s, amid a shortage of enrolling graduate students, an excess of unhappy graduate and postdoctoral stu-

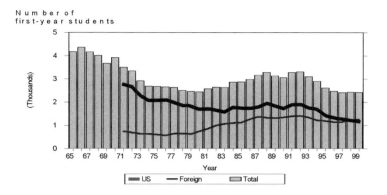

FIGURE A-4   First-year U.S. and foreign physics graduate students, 1965–1999.
SOURCE: NRC (2001).

dents, and skepticism surrounding the physics training programs available to students, physics graduate programs redesigned themselves (Feder, 2000). Several programs worked with industry, providing opportunities and internships for students. In other cases, interdisciplinary programs with business, engineering, or computer science were offered (Pimbley, 1997). Graduate programs also touted a physics education as good general training, and they began to communicate to students the realities of the physics academic world. According to some, despite these efforts and other factors, including the recent increase in federal support for physics and the development of new avenues of research, there are not enough trained and qualified individuals in the field (Freidman, 2000).

A 2001 National Research Council study, *Physics in a New Era: An Overview*, recommends that despite the many exciting frontiers in physics, changes in the recruitment and training of physicists are crucial to the future success of the field. The report notes that the number of U.S.-educated undergraduates in physics has decreased in the last 15 years, leading to an imbalance between the supply of U.S. bachelor's degree holders and the capacity of U.S. graduate programs. Physics departments have reacted by increasing the flow of students from other countries. Articles such as "Why Do They Leave Physics?" (Anderson, 1999), and "From Bear to Bull in a Decade" (Kirby et al., 2001) have described these trends. In recent years, the physics job market has opened up, and there is concern about a lack of qualified personnel to fill the available positions. The above National Research Council (2001) report confirms this, one of its strongest recommendations being to increase support for and focus on all levels of physics education.

Several factors appear to have played some part in the current trend of undergraduates not entering physics graduate programs and of physics graduates pursuing alternative careers:

• Sociological factors—The end of the Cold War, government funding cuts, industry downsizing, the influx of talented foreign scientists, and other events led to significant changes throughout science in the early 1990s and affected many young physicists who had promising scientific careers ahead of them. Graduate students who began their studies in the 1990s came to physics with their eyes wide open about their job prospects, and physics departments, as mentioned above, aware that applications for admissions were declining, began trying to sell graduate physics education as good training for many nonscientific careers. Consequently, graduate education has shifted from a kind of guild/apprenticeship model to something more akin to preprofessional training for private-sector jobs (Freidman, 2000; Feder, 2000).
• Financial factors—Financial compensation in science is significantly higher outside of academia, and industry is hiring more young people than is academia (Feder, 2000).
• Academic factors—A shift is occurring in how a physicist is recognized and credited for contributions. According to one physicist, "in lieu of scholarship, scientific achievement, and reputation, we are now assessed in terms of four so-called objective criteria: number of papers published, prestige of the journals involved, number of invited talks given, and amount of grant monies received" (Serota, 2000).
• "Horganism"—Reflecting John Horgan's philosophy that there are no new scientific laws to discover, some physicists conjecture that undergraduate students believe there is nothing left to contribute to the study of physics (Serota, 2000).

The trend of trained physicists leaving physics and of graduate students not entering physics is recognized as one of the most important issues facing the field. With regard to physics education, the National Research Council report (2001) points out that advanced undergraduate and graduate curricula should reflect physics as it is currently practiced, making appropriate connections to other areas of science, to engineering, and to schools of management. The report notes that high-quality undergraduate research opportunities are an important tool for introducing students to modern physics practice. Physics education needs to reflect the career destinations of today's students. Only a third of all physics majors pursue graduate degrees in physics, and of those who do, nearly three-quarters find permanent employment in industry. The report concludes that undergraduate and graduate curricula must satisfy the educational needs of all these students. Along with encouraging physics departments to continue to revise their curricula to be engaging and effective for a wide audience, the report's recommendations encompass two principal goals: (1) to make physics education do a better job of contributing to the scientific literacy of the general public and the training of the technical workforce, and (2) to reverse, through a better-conceived, more outward-looking curriculum, the long-term decline in the numbers of U.S. undergraduate and graduate students studying physics.

Intellectual Property

Soon after Lawrence built his first accelerator, a not-for-profit research facility, The Research Corporation, obtained the rights to the cyclotron on the understanding that Berkeley's Radiation Laboratory would continue to be a beneficiary of the corporation's policy of investing proceeds from its patents back into research at the university. Throughout World War II, accelerator laboratories across the country added their technical improvements to the machines without knowledge of whether the basic design was protected. After the war, The Research Corporation wrote a letter to all the laboratories in possession of cyclotrons requesting that they grant use of their machines without payment of royalties. Most scientists and engineers who had worked on the accelerators knew nothing of the original patent on Lawrence's cyclotron and were astonished when they received this letter. When the AEC was formed in 1946, the wartime policy of open access that had contributed greatly to the development of accelerators continued under the new agency. Since then, both law and policy have tended to grant to DOE (formerly AEC) the ownership of patentable inventions developed in its laboratories or by contractors, and to make freely available the technology of particle physics to scientists engaged in basic research. "The exemplary freedom with which high-energy physicists are accustomed to exchange information—and the speed with which the information finds application—rests on their belief that their field was never thought to have commercial or military possibilities" (Heilbron and Kevles, 1988).

CONCLUSIONS

Throughout the history of government-sponsored large-scale research projects, issues related to funding, organizing, and managing their research, and to training qualified personnel have been in constant flux, depending on how the government has allocated and reallocated the available resources, and as social needs and economic trends have changed. When funding levels have declined and acquiring research funds has become difficult, the issues have become more apparent, and a great deal of debate has ensued, but the subsequent responses have yet to stop the cycle. When funds have increased and experiments have flourished, with results of technological or economic utility, the significance of the issues has faded, and the need to create safeguards against a potentially detrimental cycle has diminished.

Academic high-energy physics has been involved with the issues of large-scale science research, as discussed throughout this paper, for over 60 years, decades longer than any other academic scientific discipline. There is consensus throughout this field, and in other fields as well, that these issues need to be addressed. The studies conducted in physics that have been cited in this paper, although few in number, have revealed that the major issues associated with large-scale research projects involve prioritizing, funding, organizing, and managing research, and educating, training, and advancing scientists. According to these few studies, one of the longest-running federally funded university-based scientific fields of the twentieth century is still grappling with almost all of these issues. There appear to be no overarching plans, solutions, or policies to serve as guidelines for large collaborations and projects. The various issues that arise during a project are quickly addressed as they appear, with no continuity.

Particle physics has followed a slightly different path from that of most of the other sciences; even within the field of physics, it has a relatively unique role. As particle physics has left the limelight, new frontiers in other areas of physics have been opening up, such as new materials; the properties and uses of fluids, plasmas, and gases; nanotechnology; and even interfaces with biology. In comparing big particle physics projects with large-scale research pursuits in biology in such areas as genomics and proteomics, one finds several differences between the fields in the definition and outcomes of their large-scale projects. Traditionally, the vast majority of expense involved in particle physics has been in building the facilities—the accelerators and detectors. Over the years, the size of the accelerators has grown of necessity from inches to miles, making them more expensive and increasingly less accessible to scientists. In contrast, technologies developed in big biology have tended to become smaller, more efficient, less expensive, and more widely available to interested scientists. Although the technologies developed in particle physics have provided a great foundation of knowledge that has led to the development of several technologies used in apparently unrelated fields, it has directly produced relatively few commercially marketable applications. Projects in biology, in contrast, have traditionally created products with tremendous commercial potential that have appealed more readily to the lay population.

While constant fluctuations in the social and economic trends and priorities of a wealthy democracy may make improving our current system for funding of scientific research challenging, continual increases in the cost of pursuing large-scale research and the competition among various areas of science for the limited funds available make addressing and resolving these issues crucial. Great utility has resulted from the pursuit of large-scale science research in an array of outcomes. It is difficult to evaluate or quantify the economic and social benefits derived from these pursuits, and little effort has been made to assess the quality or accomplishments of the various programs and approaches involved, especially in a comparative fashion. There is no doubt that the quest for scientific knowledge has provided numerous conveniences and a tremendous increase in the quality of life in less than a century. The abundance enjoyed by U.S. society has provided the means that have enabled us to engage in these pursuits. The most difficult factor has not been a lack of available resources, but the question of how to allocate those resources. This is the challenge in prioritizing research pursuits; knowing what discipline or project to fund; and deciding whether to allocate funds to a few large projects, distribute them to a large number of smaller projects, or divide them between both large and small projects. It is unfortunate that we are not able to follow Nobel Laureate Jim Watson's jest to Congress and, "only fund the breakthroughs." Until we are capable of funding only successful projects, it is important to establish helpful and realistic guidelines and policies that will ensure the ability to continue the pursuit of knowledge in the most efficient and practical way.

REFERENCES

AAAS. 2003. Guide to R&D Funding Data—Historical trends in federal R&D. Chart. Defense and Nondefense R&D, 1949–2004. http://www.aaas.org/spp/rd/guihist.htm.

AIP Center for History of Physics. 1992. AIP Study of Multi-institutional Collaborations. Phase I: High-Energy Physics. Report Number 1: Summary of Project and Findings: Project Recommendations. College Park, MD: American Institute of Physics.

Anderson PW. 1999. Why do they leave physics? *Physics Today* 52:11.

Bozeman B. 1995. Federal Laboratories: Understanding the 10,000. New York: Center for Science, Policy, and Outcomes.

Bush V. 1945a. Science: The Endless Frontier. Washington, DC: U.S. Government Printing Office.

Bush V. 1945b. As we may think. *Atlantic Monthly* 176(1):101–9.

Chollar S. 1994. Scientific alternatives: Taking roads less traveled by researchers. *Science* 265(5180)1914.

Dupree AH. 1986. Science in the Federal Government: A History of Policies and Activities. Baltimore: The Johns Hopkins University Press.

Feder T. 2000. Physics community: Physics graduate programs train students for industrial careers. *Physics Today* 53(8):39.

Flam F. 1992. Physics famine: A frenzied search for job stability. *Science* 257(5077):1726–7.

Freidman JR. 2000. Letters: More on "why do they leave physics?": Money matters, research and job opportunities. *Physics Today* 53(1):15.

Galison P, Hevly B. 1992. Big Science: The Growth of Large-scale Research. Stanford: Stanford University Press.

Goldberg S. 1995. Big Science: Atomic Bomb Research and the Beginnings of High-Energy Physics. Seattle: History of Science Society.

Green W. 1995. Two Cheers for Democracy: Science and Technology Politics. New York: Center for Science, Policy, and Outcomes.

Grice GK. 2001. The Beginning of the National Weather Service: The Signal Years (1870–1891) as Viewed by Early Weather Pioneers. Washington, DC: United States National Weather Service.

Groopman J. 2001. The Thirty Years' War. New York: The New Yorker.

Heilbron JL, Kevles DJ. 1988. Finding a policy for mapping and sequencing the human genome: Lessons from the history of particle physics. *Minerva* 29:299–314.

Heilbron JL, Seidel RW, Wheaton BR. 1981. Lawrence and his laboratory: Nuclear science at Berkeley. *LBL News Magazine* 6(3).

Institute of Food and Agricultural Sciences (IFAS). 2000. Land Grants: Events Leading to the Establishment of Land-grant Universities. Gainesville: University of Florida.

Kevles DJ. 1995. *The Physicists: The History of a Scientific Community in Modern America*. 4th ed. Cambridge, MA: Harvard University Press.

Killian JR. 1982. A Brief Analysis of University Research and Development Efforts Relating to National Security, 1940–1980. Washington, DC: National Academy Press.

King J. 1991. Many top researchers are disenchanted with big science. *The Scientist* 5(1):13.

Kirby K, Czujko R, Mulvey P. 2001. The physics job market: From bear to bull in a decade. *Physics Today* 54(4):36–41.

Kolb A, Hoddeson L. 1992. The Mirage of the World Accelerator for World Peace and the Origins of the SSC, 1953–1983. Batavia, IL: Fermi National Accelerator Laboratory. FERMILAB-Pub-92/375.

National Archives and Records Administration. Records of the Coast and Geodetic Survey (1807–1965). Record Group 23.

National Archives and Records Administration. Records of the Office of Naval Research (ONR).

National Institutes of Health (NIH). 2001. History of the NIH. Bethesda, MD: NIH.

National Research Council. 1995. Setting Priorities for Space Research: An Experiment in Methodology. Washington, DC: National Academy Press.

National Research Council. Board on Physics and Astronomy. 2001. Physics in a New Era: An Overview. Washington, DC: National Academy Press.

Naval Research Laboratory. 2001. NRL History. Washington, DC: Naval Research Laboratory.

Office of Science and Technology Policy. 2001. About OSTP. Washington, DC.

Old BS. 1982. Return on Investment in Basic Research—Exploring a Methodology. National Academy of Engineering. Washington, DC.

Old BS, The Bird Dogs. 1961. The evolution of the Office of Naval Research. *Physics Today* 14(8):30–35.

Pimbley JM. 1997. Physicists in Finance. *Physics Today* 50(1):42.

Price DJ. 1963. *Little Science, Big Science*. New York and London: Columbia University Press.

Price DK. 1962. The scientific establishment. *Science* 136:1099–1106.

Public Broadcasting Service (PBS). 1999. Establishment of the United States Geological Survey, 1879. *The American Experience: Lost in the Grand Canyon*. Alexandria, VA: PBS.

Rabbitt MC. 2000. The United States Geological Survey: 1879–1989. *USGS Circular 1050*. Washington, DC: United States Geological Survey.

Rettig R. 1977. *Cancer Crusade: The Story of the National Cancer Act of 1971*. Princeton, NJ: Princeton University Press.

Rosenberg CE. 1997. *No Other Gods: On Science and American Social Thought*. Revised and expanded edition. Baltimore, MD: Johns Hopkins University Press.

Serota RA. 2000. Letters: More on "why do they leave physics?": Money matters, research and job opportunities. *Physics Today* 53(1):75.

Smith CHL. 1998. What's the Use of Basic Science? Why Governments Must Support Basic Science. Geneva, Switzerland: CERN.

Tobias S. 1994. Unemployment blues: A report from the field. *Science* 265(5180):1931–32.

U.S. Congressional Yellow Book. 2001. Washington, DC: United States Government Printing Office.

U.S. Department of Energy. 2001. Inside the DOE: Our History. Washington, DC: Department of Energy.

U.S. National Oceanic and Atmospheric Administration. The Coast and Geodetic Survey Annual Reports 1844–1919 bibliography.

Universities Research Association. 2001. About URA, Inc. Washington, DC: Universities Research Association.

Weinberg A. 1961. Impact of large-scale science on the United States. *Science* 134:161–164.

Weinberg A. 1967. Reflections on Big Science. Cambridge: The MIT Press. Pg. 39.

Wilson RR. 1975. A world laboratory and world peace. *Physics Today* 18(11).

Index

A

Academic research, *see* Universities and colleges
Adams Act, 223
Administration, *see* Organization and management
Advanced Photon Source, 73-74
Advisory committees, 2, 42, 44, 48, 51, 57, 60, 61, 78-79, 86, 92, 100-101, 134, 193, 233, 234-235, 240, 243, 248, 256
   intellectual property, 186-187, 190
Advocacy and advocacy groups
   Human Genome Project, 31, 33
   NIH funding, 95
AIDS, *see* HIV/AIDS
Alliance for Cellular Signaling, 55-56
American Association for the Advancement of Science, 221, 244
American Institute of Physics, 246-256 (passim)
Animal models
   cancer, 41, 46, 50-52, 114
   genomics, 28, 34, 36, 40, 121-122
Antitrust regulations, 172-173, 174
Applied Biosystems Incorporated, 37

Argonne National Laboratory, 73-74
Assessment, *see* Evaluation and assessment
Association of University Technology Managers, 175
Atomic Energy Act, 240-241
Atomic Energy Commission, 232, 233, 240-241
   see also Department of Energy

B

Bayh-Dole Act, 28(n.2), 47, 116, 163, 166, 175, 188, 189
Bermuda Rules, *see* International Strategy Meeting on Human Genome Sequencing
Best practices, 4, 194
Bioinformatics
   see also Databases
   cancer research, 23
   cooperative agreements, 122-123
   definition of large-scale research, 17, 23
   Human Genome Project, 34, 35
   Human Proteome Organization, 71
   small- *vs* large-scale research, 2, 18